Community Health Nursing for GNM (1st Year)

Community Health Nursing for GNM (1st Year)

Solved Papers with Important Theory (2016–2004)

As per INC Syllabus

Third Edition

Most Authentic and Updated Solved Question Papers

Poonam Sharda
Post Basic BSc Nursing
Baba Farid University of Health Sciences
Faridkot, Punjab, India

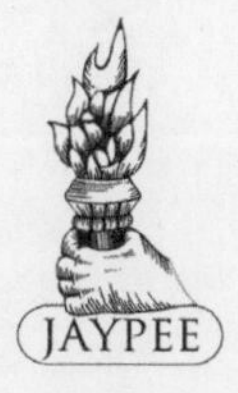

The Health Sciences Publisher

New Delhi | London | Panama

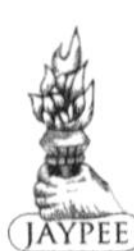

Jaypee Brothers Medical Publishers (P) Ltd

Headquarters

Jaypee Brothers Medical Publishers (P) Ltd.
4838/24, Ansari Road, Daryaganj
New Delhi 110 002, India
Phone: +91-11-43574357
Fax: +91-11-43574314
Email: jaypee@jaypeebrothers.com

Overseas Offices

J.P. Medical Ltd.
83, Victoria Street, London
SW1H 0HW (UK)
Phone: +44-20 3170 8910
Fax: +44-(0)20 3008 6180
Email: info@jpmedpub.com

Jaypee-Highlights Medical Publishers Inc.
City of Knowledge, Bld. 235, 2nd Floor, Clayton
Panama City, Panama
Phone: +1 507-301-0496
Fax: +1 507-301-0499
Email: cservice@jphmedical.com

Jaypee Brothers Medical Publishers (P) Ltd.
Bhotahity, Kathmandu, Nepal
Phone: +977-9741283608
Email: kathmandu@jaypeebrothers.com

Jaypee Brothers Medical Publishers (P) Ltd.
17/1-B, Babar Road, Block-B, Shaymali
Mohammadpur, Dhaka-1207
Bangladesh
Mobile: +08801912003485
Email: jaypeedhaka@gmail.com

Website: www.jaypeebrothers.com
Website: www.jaypeedigital.com

Community Health Nursing for GNM (1st Year)

First Edition: 2013

Second Edition: 2014

Third Edition: **2017**

ISBN: 978-93-86322-20-3

Printed at

Dedicated to

My Parents

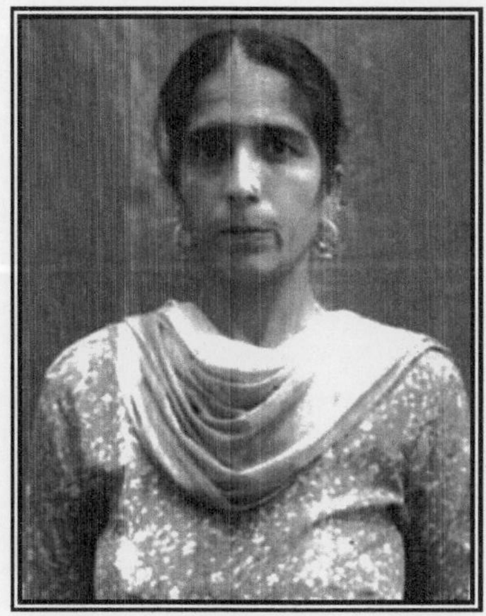

Smt Raj Rani

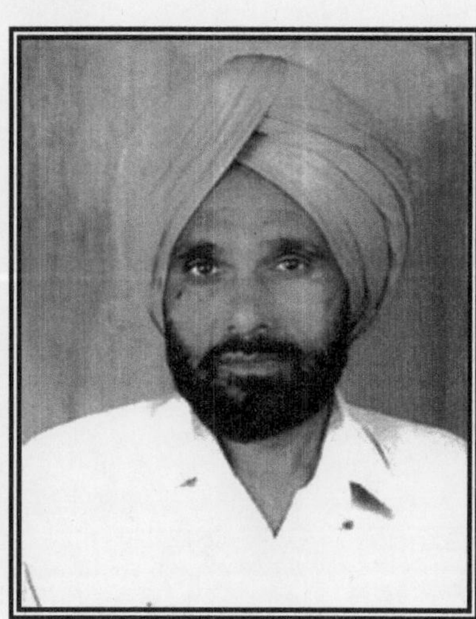

Sh Rajkumar

Preface

It is matter of great pride to present Nursing Solved Question Papers for the first year students of General Nursing and Midwifery (GNM).

As a student, I found difficulty in getting an authentic question bank during my exams. However, there were few books available in the market but they were not having the authentic questions with relevant answers so, I have compiled this question bank which appeared in Baba Farid University of Punjab as per INC regulations.

Community Health Nursing for GNM is written with great attention and concentration keeping in mind the basic requirements of Ist year nursing students. It contains solved question papers of Community Health Nursing with detailed explanations and important theory given at the beginning of every subject.

I am sure that this book will prove really beneficial to nursing students and will enable them to prepare well for their examination even without books.

Poonam Sharda

Acknowledgments

I am thankful to the God who strengthens me in each and every second in all my work by showing His blessings abundantly through various resources which helped me in accomplishment of the entire task in my life.

My sincere heartfelt thanks to my respected parents Sh Rajkumar and Smt Raj Rani for their help, support and encouragement given to me to achieve this level. Without their help this would not have been possible for me to complete this project.

My sincere thanks goes to Jaypee Brothers Medical Publishers for giving me great opportunity to publish this book.

INC Syllabus

COMMUNITY HEALTH NURSING I

Hours: 80

COURSE DESCRIPTION

This course is designed to help students gain an understanding of the concept of community health in order to introduce them to the wider horizons of rendering nursing services in a community set-up, both in urban and rural areas.

GENERAL OBJECTIVE

Upon completion of this course, the students will be able to:

- Describe the concept of health, community health and community health nursing
- State the principles of epidemiology and epidemiological method of community health nursing practice
- Explain the various services provided to the community and the role of the nurse
- Demonstrate skills to practice effective nursing care of the individuals and families in the clinics as well as in their homes, using scientific principles.

COURSE CONTENT

Unit I: Introduction to Community Health and Community Health Nursing:

- Health and disease
- Community, community health, community health nursing
- Dimensions of health
- Health determinants
- Indicators of health levels of health care
- **Primary health care:** Elements and principles Nurse's role in primary health care
- Health for all by 2000 AD

- Evolution and development of community health nursing in India and its present concept
- Differences between institutional and community health nursing
- Community health team functioning
- Philosophy, goals, objectives and principles of community health nursing practice
- Qualities and functions of a community health nurse.

Unit II: Community Health Nursing Process

- Concepts and definition
- Importance of the community health nursing process
- Steps of the process: Community identification, population composition, health and allied resources, community assessment, planning and conducting community health nursing care services.

Unit III: Health Assessment

- Characteristics of healthy individual
- Identification of deviation from normal health.

Unit IV: Principles of Epidemiology and Epidemiological Methods

- Definition and aims of epidemiology
- Basic tools of measurement in epidemiology
- Uses of epidemiology
- Disease cycle
- Spectrum of disease
- Levels of prevention of disease
- Disease transmission-direct and indirect
- Immunity
- Immunizing agents and immunization schedule
- Control of infectious diseases
- Disinfection.

Unit V: Family Health Nursing Care

- Concept, goals, objectives, family as a unit of health family health care services
- Family health and nursing care process—family health assessment, family care plan
- Family health services—maternal, child care and family welfare services

- Roles and function of a community health nurse in family health services
- Family health records.

Unit VI: Family Health Care Settings

- Home visiting
- Purposes
- Principles
- Planning and evaluation
- Bag technique
- Clinic
- Purposes
- Types of clinics and their functions
- Setting up of various clinics
- Functions of health personnel in these clinics.

Unit VII: Referral Systems

Unit VIII: Records and Reports

- Types of records
- Uses of records
- Essential requirements of records
- Cumulative records
- Design of cards/records.

Unit IX: Minor Ailments

- Classification
- Early detection and management
- Standing instructions/orders.

ENVIRONMENTAL HYGIENE

Hours: 20

COURSE DESCRIPTION

This course is designed to help students acquire the concept of health, understanding of the principles of environmental health and its relation to nursing in health and disease.

GENERAL OBJECTIVES

Upon completion of this course, the students will be to:

- Describe the concept of environmental health
- Describe the principles of environmental health
- Demonstrate skills to apply these principles in the pursing care of the patients/clients as well as in their own healthy living
- Describe the environmental health hazards and health problems of the country and services available to meet these.

COURSE CONTENT

Unit I: Introduction

- Components of environment
- Importance of environmental health.

Unit II: Environmental Factors Contributing to Healthy Water

- Safe and wholesome water
- Uses of water
  - Water pollution
  - Waterborne diseases
  - Water purification.

Air

- Air pollution
- Prevention and control of air pollution.

Waste

- Refuse
- Excreta
- Sewage
- Health hazards of these wastes
- Collection removal and disposal of these wastes.

Housing

- Site
- Basic amenities
- Types and standard of ventilation

- Requirements of good lighting
- Natural and artificial lighting.

Noise

- Sources of noise
- Community noise levels
- Effects of noise
- Noise control.

Arthropods of Public Health Importance

- Mosquitoes, housefly, sandfly, human louse, ratfleas, etc.
- Rodents
- Control measures for these arthropods.

Unit III: Community Organization to Promote Environmental Health

Levels and types of agencies: National, state, local, government, voluntary and social agencies.

HEALTH EDUCATON AND COMMUNICATION SKILLS

Hours: 20

COURSE DESCRIPTION

This course is designed to help students acquire the concept of health education and understanding of the principles underlying health education in order to develop an ability to communicate effectively with the patients, community, health team members and others.

GENERAL OBJECTIVES

Upon completion of this course, the students will be able to:

- Describe the concept of health education, communication skills, audio-visual education agencies
- Identify and utilize opportunities for health education planned and incidental
- Communicate effectively with others.

COURSE CONTENT

Unit I: Introduction

- Concept, definition, aims and objectives of health education
- Process of change/modification of health behavior
- Opportunities of health education in hospital and community
- Scope of health education
- Levels and approaches of health education
- Principles of health education
- Nurse's role as health educator.

Unit II: Communication Skills

- Definition of communication
- Purposes of communication
- Process of communication
- Barriers of communication and establishment of successful communication
- Types of communication
- Importance and art of observing and listening in communication.

Unit III: Methods and Media of Health Education

- Methods of health education
- Types of media (AV Aids)
- Advantages and limitations of each
- Preparation and uses of simple aids.

Unit IV: Health Education Agencies

- National
- State
- District
- Local.

NUTRITION

Hours: 30

COURSE DESCRIPTION

This course is designed to help students understand that nutrition is an integral component of health, since nutrition play a vital role in the growth, development and maintenance of the body.

GENERAL OBJECTIVES

Upon completion of this course, the students will be able to:

- Describe the principles of nutrition and dietetics and its relationship to the human body in health and disease
- Describe the common foods in health and disease
- Apply knowledge in the promotion of health and in the care of sick
- Demonstrate skills in selection, preparation and preservation of foods.

COURSE CONTENT

Unit I: Introduction

- Changing concepts—food habits and customs
- Relationship of nutrition to health.

Unit II: Classification of Food

Classification by Origin

- Food of animal origin
- Food of vegetable origin.

Contents

Important Theory

- **Community health:** According to WHO `Community Health' refers to the health status of the members of the community, to the problems affecting their health, and to the totality of health care provided to the community.
- **Community:** Community is a human population, living within limited geographical area and sharing a common life.

  Or

  A community is a network of human relationships, it is the place where our home is located, children are educated, sick people are treated and individual basic needs and desires are met.
- **Health:** According to WHO `Health' is defined as `It is the complete status of physical, mental, social and spiritual well-being and not merely an absence of disease or infirmity.'
- **Pasteurization:** According to WHO `Pasteurization' has been defined as the heating of milk to such temperatures for such periods of time as are required to destroy any pathogens, that may be present] while causing minimal changes in the composition, flavor and nutrition value.
- **Safe and wholesome water:** It means a water which is free from micro-organisms and chemical substance, has good taste and is fit for domestic use.
- **Incubation period:** It is time interval between entry of micro-organism of disease-causing agent in the body and occurrence of signs and symptoms.
- **Sewage:** It is defined as the water from a community, houses, street, washing, factories and industries which contains solid and liquid excreta.
- **Ventilation:** It may be defined as exchange of air between outdoors and indoors.
- **Immunity:** It is the ability of body to fight against infection.

  Or

  Immunity is the ability of body to fight, destroy and eliminate antigenic material.
- **Disinfection:** Killing of infectious agents outside the human body by direct exposure to chemical or physical agents.

- **Fomites:** Fomites are articles other than food and drinking which are contaminated by infectious agents such as pencil, toys, drinking glass, etc.
- **Nutrition:** Nutrition is intake of food considered in relation to the body's dietary needs.
- **Balanced diet:** Balanced diet is the one which consists of all the required nutrients in correct or adequate amount for proper maintenance and regulation of the body functions.
- **Pandemic:** (Pan = all, demos = people) so, pandemic means disease spread from country to country or over the whole worlds for example AIDS, swine flu, etc.
- **Epidemic:** (Epi = upon, demos = people) an outbreak of disease in a community in excess of "normal expectation," derived from common source.
- **Eradication:** Termination of all transmission of infection by examination of the infection agents through surveillance.
- **Preservation:** It is a technique in which variety of foods are stored for a long period.
- **Cross-infection:** It means infection transmitted from one to another individuals infected with different pathogenic organisms.
- **Weaning:** It is supplementary food, e.g. kheer, suzi, milk, juice, fruits, boiled vegetables, etc. which start from 6 months of age with breast-feed.
- **Immunization:** The process which increases the resistance of a person to a particular infection by artificial means is called immunization.
- **Disease:** Any deviation from normal well-being] is called disease.
- **Infection:** The entry and development of disease-producing agent in the body is known as infection.
- **Cold chain:** It is a system of transporting and storing vaccines at the recommended temperatures.
- **IMR (Infant mortality rate):** Infant mortality rate is defined as the number of infant deaths or number of deaths under one year of age per 1000 live births in one year.
- **Motivation:** It is inner force which drives (directs) an individual to do some actions.
- **Rehabilitation:** The process of restoring a person's ability to live and work as normally as possible after any illness and injury.
- **Refuse:** Refuse is discarded waste matter, the term now applied to refuse from houses, street sweepings, commercial, industrial and agricultural operations. Refuse is also called "litters".

- **Communicable disease:** The disease which spreads from one person to another's is called communicable disease, for example, tuberculosis (TB).
- **Vital statistics:** Vital statistics have been defined as the facts, systematically collected and compiled in numerical form, related to vital event.
- **Psychology:** It is a study of human behavior, means how people behave. It is wrong concept that psychology is a study of mind.
- **Chlorination:** It is a process of mixing chlorine in the water for purification.
- **Personality:** Personality means quality of human behavior, for example his mode of thinking, attitude, interest, belief, capacities and philosophy of life, his physical, mental and emotional characteristics constitude his personality.
- **Primary heath care:** Primary health care is essential health care made universally accessible to individual and acceptable to them through their full participation and at a cost that the community and country can afford.
- **Crude death rate:** It is defined as the number of deaths per 1000 population per year in a given community.

IMPORTANT QUESTIONS AND ANSWERS

1. Mention difference between community health nursing and hospital nursing services.

Ans.

Hospital nurse	Community health nurse
• She follows orders.	• She observes, thinks, decides and acts.
• Services are provided according to demand of patient.	• Services provided to all community.
• She commands hospital administration, patients and family.	• Family is in command and people can accept or reject advice of health workers.
• Focuses on curative services.	• The focus of planning is preventive and promotive services.
• She provides care in hospital setting.	• She visits the house and assesses the needs of people.
• She provides care in hospital with all techniques of hospital.	• She carries out simple procedure in the home of people.

2. What are the principles of primary health care?

Ans. There are five principles of PHC.

- **Equitable distribution:** The first principle of primary health care is equitable distribution. The health services should reach to all people and give attention to needy and vulnerable group.
- **Community involvement:** Involve the community people in planning, implementation and evaluation of health services. So, that people get more effectiveness from health services.

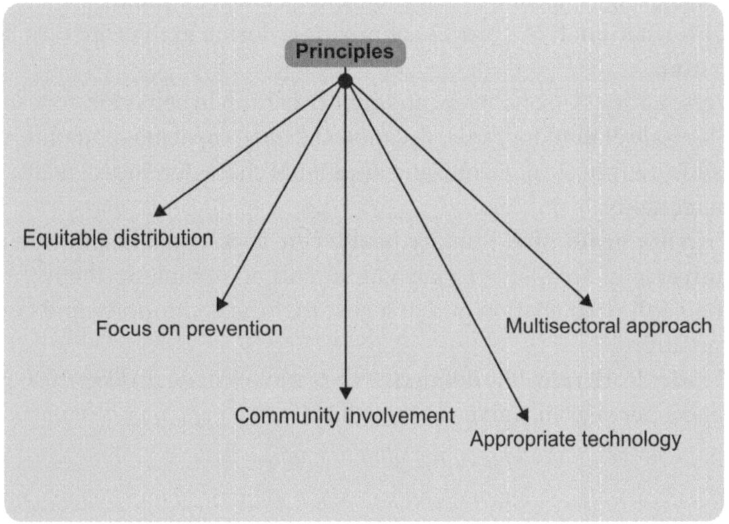

- **Appropriate technology:** Attentions hould be made on the methods or material, which are socially acceptable and affordable by all.
- **Prevention:** It is very important principle of primary health care that focuses on prevention. For this, all elements of primary health care followed.
- **Multisectrol approach:** For achievement of better heath, it requires joint efforts of other health-related sectors such as agriculture, education and social welfare.

3. What were the specific goals set-up by national health policy to be achieved by 2000 AD.

Ans. Reduction of infant mortality rate from the present level then 125 to below 60 by the year 2000AD:

- To raise the expectation of life from 52 years to 64 by the year 2000 AD.
- To reduce crude death rate from 12 per 1000 population to 9 by the year 2000 AD.
- To achieve a net reproduction rate of one by the year 2000 AD.

- To reduce the crude birth rate from 32 per 1,000 population to 21 per 1,000 by the year 2000 AD.

4. What are the name of national program started to solve the problem, and role of a nurse in these programs?

Ans.

- National malaria eradication program
- National filaria control program
- National TB control program
- National water supply and sanitation program
- Expanded program on immunization
- National family planning program
- National program for prevention of blindness
- National AIDS control program.

ROLE OF NURSE IN THESE PROGRAMS

Nurse plays an important role in all national programs. She plays the following roles:

- **Early detection:** She plays a role in early detection of all communicable diseases and provides appropriate treatment.
- **Health education:** In this, she has to give health education to the people on different topics, which are related to communicable diseases, their modes of transmission and about preventive measures, etc.
- **Supervision:** She supervises the other health worker who helps in providing of health care services.
- **Coordination:** She coordinates with other heath personnel for the success of these programmers.
- **Research and evaluation:** She participates in all research programs which are working against communicable disease and evaluates the progress of all national programs to find out the effectiveness.

These are main roles of a nurse in national programs.

5. What are the principles of home visiting?

Ans. Home visiting should be made according to the need of the people:

- It should be part of planned visiting program.
- Collect all background information related to family and community in which include size of family, occupation, income, religion, custom and cultures.
- Identify the health problems of the family.
- Use safe technical skills and nursing procedures.
- In health teaching, be sure of what you discuss.

- The approach with community should be kind for gaining confidence.

6. Explain the principles of health education.

Ans.
- **Interest:** If the people are not interested, they will not learn. To make the education effective, it is essential that education should be according to interest of people and need of people.
- **Participation:** It is key principle of health education. Provide opportunities to people for participation by discussion because personal involvement leads to personal acceptance.
- **Comprehension:** The teaching should be provided according to understanding capacity of people. Use local and simple language. Strange and difficult words should be avoided.
- **Motivation:** Try to motivate the people to accept new ideas.
- **Communication:** Use simple and local language for education, not use new and difficult words.
- **Reinforcement:** Few people do not learn all new things in single period. Repetition, at intervals, is necessary.
- **Learning by doing:** Focus on actions because:
  - If I hear, I forget
  - If I see, I remember
  - If I do, I know.
- **Good human relationship:** The health educators must be kind and sympathetic; people must accept him as real friend. Good relationship is essential for health education.

7. Explain the components of communication.

Ans. Components of communication are:

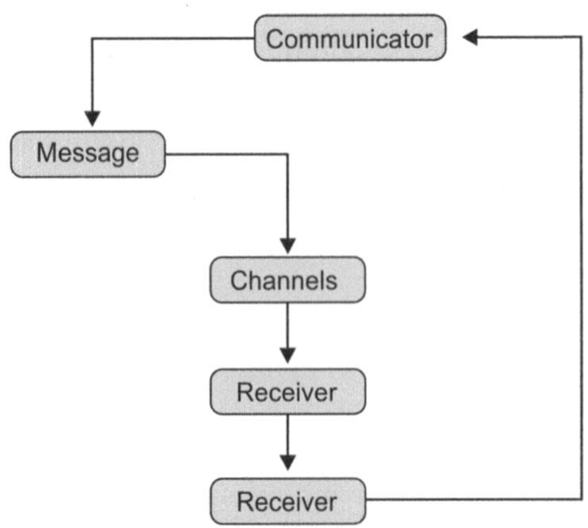

- **Communicator:** Who sends the message according to the wishes of audience, with objective and in clear form.
- **Message:** It is piece of information, which is communicated by communicator. A good message must be objective, clear, understandable, accurate, timely and according to need.
- **Channels:** These are TV, radio, books, newspapers, etc. used by sender to communicate the information.
- **Audience or receiver:** Audience may be total population or target group, who receive information.
- **Feedback:** It is response which is given by audience or receiver to sender.

8. What are the levels of prevention?

Ans. There are three levels of prevention:

1. Primary prevention
2. Secondary prevention
3. Tertiary prevention

PRIMARY PREVENTION

Primary prevention can be defined as `action' taken prior to onset of disease, which removes the possibility of disease will ever occur.

The specific interventions are:

- Health promotion
- Specific protection.

Health Promotion

We can prevent a number of diseases by promoting health, for example, typhoid, fever, cholera, TB, etc.

Specific Protection

By specific protection, we prevent some specific diseases, for example, by immunization (TB diphtheria, pertussis tetanus, polio, measles), etc.

SECONDARY PREVENTION

It means the action which stops the progress of disease and prevents complications. The intervention includes:

- Early diagnosis
- Adequate treatment.

Diagnosis and appropriate treatment help to stop the disease progress. It is more effective in case of STD (sexual transmitted disease), etc.

TERTIARY PREVENTION

When diseases progress and reach at high level, if it is still possible to prevent, that is called tertiary prevention.

This includes:

- Disability limitation
- Rehabilitation.

Recover the patient from illness and restore body function at normal level.

9. What are the functions of a community health nurse?

Ans. Functions of a CHN classified into following headings:

1. Administration
2. Communication
3. Nursing
4. Teaching
5. Research

ADMINISTRATION

The nurses is responsible for the day assignment of the nursing staff and supervises them. She acts as a leader. She is responsible in planning, implementation and evaluation of nursing care plan at PHC and sub centers.

COMMUNICATION

This involves ability to maintain good working relationship with members of the health team, other agencies and the community. She participates with the staff in community meetings.

NURSING

She provides comprehensive nursing care to individuals and families. It includes maternal and child care, nutrition and family planning.

TEACHING

She provides education to individual and group by using simple teaching aids. She gives training to dais, health workers and students, etc.

RESEARCH

She participates in all research activities related to health and utilization (use) of the existing nursing services.

10. What are the uses of records?

Ans.
- Effective means of communication. Records are those methods used to communicate information to another health worker.
- It helps in providing best possible service to the individual, family and community.
- It can be save time, effort and money. Because once maintained, record can be used anytime.
- It helps the health worker to organize his work and make the most effective use of his time.
- Records is useful in research. It provides necessary data for the research activity.
- Records can be useful in health education, for example, growth charts, etc.

11. What are the methods of refuse disposal?

BURNING

The best method is burning or incineration. Hospital refuse best disposed by burning. But before burning, remove glasses and tin materials.

DUMPING

It is simple method of refuse disposal by dumping in low-lying area, where after some time, it changes in mannure and it is very useful for vegetation.

CONTROLLED TIPPING

In this method, make 3 feet depth pit and the refuse is disposed in this pit. After 3 to 6 months, it changes in manure by bacterial action. At the end of 6 months, open the pit and remove manure for agriculture use.

COMPOSTING

When disposed human excreta along with refuse in 3 feet deep pit, is called composting. Fill the pit with alternate layers of excreta and refuse.

12. Write down national immunization schedule.

Ans.

S. No.	Age	Vaccine	Dose	Route	Prevention from
1.	At birth within 72 hrs	BCG dose of OPV	0.1 ml 2–3 doses	I/d Orally	TB, Polio (Tuberculosis)
2.	1 ½ months	DPT+OPV+ Hep B	0.5 ml, 2 drops, 0.5 ml	IM, Orally, IM	Diphtheria persuing tetanus Hep B, Polio
3.	2 ½ months	DPT + OPV + Hep B	Same as above	Same as above	Same as above
4.	3 ½ months	DPT + OPV	0.5 ml, 2 drops	IM, orally	Same as above
5.	4 ½ months	OPV (4th dose)	2 drops	Orally	Polio
6.	5 ½ months	OPV (5th dose)	2 drops	Orally	Polio
7.	7 ½ months	Hepatitis B (3rd dose)	0.5 ml	IM	Hepatitis
8.	9 months	Measles + syp Vitamin A	0.5 ml, 1 lac IV	S/C orally	Measles
9.	15 months	MMR	0.5 ml	S/C	Measles mumps rubella
10.	18 months	DPT + OPV	0.5 ml 2 drops	IM orally	Diphtheria pertussis tetanus polio
11.	5 yrs	DPT + OPV	0.5 ml 2 drops	IM orally	Same as above
12.	10 yrs	TT	0.5 ml	IM	Tetanus
13.	16 yrs	TT	0.5 ml	IM	Tetanus

Abbreviations

OPV Oral polio vaccine
TT Tetanus toxoid
S/C Subcutaneous
IM Intramuscular
Orally By mouth
T/d Intradermally
MMR Measles, mumps, rubella

For Pregnant Women

Early in pregnancy	TT-1 dose
One month after TT-I	TT-2

13. What are the indicators of health assessment?

Ans.

Indicators used to fix out the health status.

Uses of Indicators

- Indicators are required/used to measure the health status of community.
- To compare the health status of one country with other country.
- For assessment of health care needs.
- For monitoring and evaluation of heath service activities and programs.

Characteristics of Indicators

- It should be valid.
- It should be reliable.
- It should be specific.
- It should be feasible.
- It should be relevant.

Main Indicators of Health are:

- Mortality indicators
- Morbidity indicators
- Disability rates
- Nutritional status indicators
- Health care delivery indicators
- Utilization rates
- Indicators of social and mental health
- Environmental indicators
- Socioeconomic indicators
- Health policy indicators
- Indicators of quality of life
- Other indicators.

14. What are the characteristics of sanitary latrines?

CHARACTERISTICS OF SANITARY LATRINES

- There is no need for the services of sweeper for daily removal of night soil.
- The excreta does not pollute the ground or surface water.

- Feces is not exposed to flies, rodents, and animals such as pigs.
- The excreta does not create dirt and bad smell.

15. What are the major causes of death under-five years of age?

ENVIRONMENTAL CAUSE

- Lack of safe drinking water
- Lack of basic sanitation
- Overcrowding
- Inadequate sanitary living condition
- Pollution of water, food and air.

SOCIOECONOMIC CAUSE

- Poverty
- Illiteracy
- Ignorance
- Customs and traditions
- Inadequate nutrition
- Lack of personal hygiene
- Rapid population growth.

OTHERS

- Uneven development of health care services and nursing care.
- Inadequate primary health care.

16. What are the aims of school health services?

AIMS OF SCHOOL HEALTH SERVICES

- To increase health awareness among children to a level where they can treat health as a personal, family and community issue.
- To promote growth and development of school children through health supervision, health care and nutrition program.
- To prevent and control communicable diseases.
- To promote healthy school living so that the school child may develop favorable attitude towards health.
- To promote good healthy habits in children.
- To facilitate early diagnosis and treatment of diseases in school children.
- To promote interest of students in individual and community health activities.

17. What are the elements of primary health care?

Ans. According to Alma Atta declaration, primary health care includes at least 7 elements:

- Education of the people about health problems and methods of preventing and controlling them.
- Promotion of food supply and proper nutrition.
- Adequate supply of safe water and basic sanitation.
- Maternal and child health care and family planning.
- Immunization against major infectious diseases.
- Prevention and control of locally endemic diseases.
- Provision of essential drugs.

18. What are the roles of a nurse in primary health care?

Ans. A WHO expert committee in 1984 defined the role of a nurse in PHC:

- Assessing the health status of individuals and communities.
- She works with population, community, family and at individual level. She focuses on maintaining and promotion of health.
- Providing complete care including the treatment of emergencies and making rafferrals.
- Maintaining epidemiological survey.
- The community health nurse works in school, home, clinic setupss.
- She provides treatment and supervises health workers.
- Collaborating with other health and development agencies.
- Monitoring progress in primary health care.

19. What are the modes of disease transmission?

Ans.

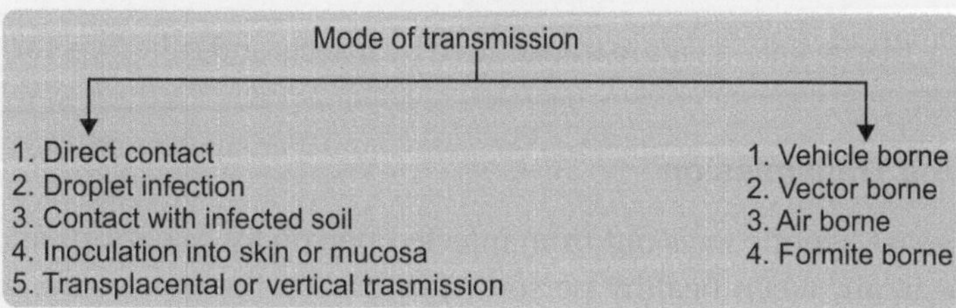

DIRECT

Direct Contact

The disease which spreads from person to person by kissing, sexual contact is called direct contact. AIDS, scabies, leprosy are examples of diseases.

Droplet Infection

The infection which spreads from fine drops released by infected person by sneezing, coughing, etc. is called droplet infection, e.g. TB, common cold, diphtheria, whooping cough spread through this method.

Contact with Infected Soil

Some disease agents are acquired by dirty soil. For example, tetanus, hookworm, etc.

Inoculation into Skin or Mucosa

The disease agent may be inoculated directly into the skin, e.g. rabies virus by dog-bite, hepatitis by contaminated needles and syringes.

Transplacental Transmission

Disease agent transferred from mother to fetus through placenta is called transplacental transmission, for example, AIDS.

INDIRECT TRANSMISSION

Vehicle borne Transmission

The chief vehicles are water, milk or food, blood, serum, plasma, etc. The diseases transmitted by these are enteric fever, food poisoning by food and water. Hepatitis 'B' is transmitted through blood products.

Vector borne Transmission

Malaria, filaria, kala-azar are transmitted by insects and called vector-borne diseases.

Airborne Transmission

The disease agent comes out from infected person by fine drops and start to float in air, when healthy person takes breath, the inhales the disease agent and develops infection. Tuberculosis, common cold, measles are, examples of airborne disease.

Fomite borne Transmission

The disease spread by the articles other than food and drink, which are contaminated by patient is called fomiteborne disease. It plays an important role in indirect transmission of disease articles such as pencil, books, door handle, clothes, etc.

20. Mention the aims and objectives of underfive clinic.

Ans. Aims and objectives of underfive clinics set out in symbol:

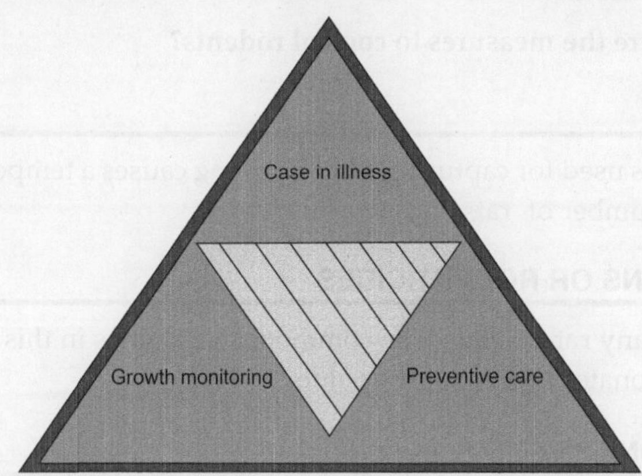

CARE IN ILLNESS

The apex of the triangle represents a care and treatment of sick children. Care in illness can be provided by nurses; for that they are given proper training and assigned duties.

PREVENTIVE CARE

- **Immunization:** Immunization is birth right of every child. It is the aim of health for all 2000 AD. Provide immunization to all children against six killer diseases.
- **Nutritional surveillance:** To check the nutritional status of every child, and working to prevent from nutritional deficiency disease. ICDS in India has taken up supplementary feeding of children below 6 years of age.
- **Health check-up:** The child health card provides a checklist for these examinations.
- **Oral rehydration:** The mothers are taught about oral rehydration therapy.
- **Health teaching:** Around the symbol is a border, it represents health teaching. It is essential part of services.

GROWTH MONITORING

One of the basic activities of the under-five clinic is growth monitoring. In which includes height and weight of child, measured periodically and recorded on health card.

21. What are the measures to control rodents?

TRAPPING

This device is used for capturing rats. Trapping causes a temporary reduction in the number of rats.

RAT POISONS OR RODENTICIDES

There are many rat poisons. The commonly used ones in this country are barium carbonates and zinc phosphide.

FUMIGATION

Cyanogas is used for fumigation. Trained persons are required for fumigation.

IMPROVEMENT OF SANITATION

Rat requires the things, food, water and shelter, if these three things are properly stopped red, rats are naturally eliminated.

- Proper storage of food
- Make a rat proof building
- Proper disposal of garbage.

22. What are the components of school health services?

HEALTH APPRAISAL

It includes periodic medical examinations or observation of children by class teacher. Teacher is in a unique position to carry out the daily inspection. The nurse identifies the children who needs medical attention.

Unusually flushed face, any rash or spots, sore throat, cough, sneezing nausea, vomiting, headache, chills, fever, etc.

TREATMENT AND FOLLOW-UP

Only health check-up is not enough, also give appropriate treatment and follow-up. The required number of specialists should be employed in the school health services.

SCHOOL SANITATION

The school should be a model of good sanitation. There should be adequate, safe drinking water facilities, one urinal for 60 students and one sanitary latrine for 100 students.

IMMUNIZATION

The school offers excellent opportunities for immunization of children against the locally endemic disease.

NUTRITIONAL SERVICES

The community health nurse administers the following nutritional services.

- Mid-day meal
- Vitamin A prophylaxis program.

FIRST AID

In every school, a fully equipped first aid box should be at hand. The emergencies commonly met within school are:

- Accidents
- Injuries
- Medical emergencies such as pain, fainting, etc.

HEALTH EDUCATION

Health education is provided on hygiene of skin, hair, teeth and clothing, importance of exercise, sleep and nutrition.

SCHOOL HEALTH RECORDS

The health record of each student should be properly maintained. It contains identification data, name, date of birth, address, past medical history, records of services provided, etc.

23. What are the points of the barriers of communication?

Ans. These may be:

- Physiological : Difficulties in hearing
- Psychological : Emotional disturbance, nervousness, fear anxiety, etc.
- Environmental : Noise, invisibility
- Cultural : Customs, beliefs, religion, attitudes and levels of knowledge.

24. What are the methods of sewage purification?

Ans. There are 2 stages in purification–primary and secondary.

PRIMARY PREVENTION

- **Screening:** The sewage first passes through metal screen where there is removal of all floating objects.
- **Grit chamber:** The water next passes from grit chamber, in this, all solids and sand sattle down.
- **Primary sedimentation:** Now water enters into huge tank and spends 6 to 8 hours in primary sedimentation tank. All sludge settles down which is removed is pumped into sludge tank.

SECONDARY TREATMENT

Now water enters into secondary tank and starts aerobic oxidation process:

- **Trickling filter method:** The effluent from primary sedimentation tank to trickling filter. It is bed of stone 4 to 8 feet deep and 6 to 100 feet diameter. In this way bacteria form zoological layer which help in purification of sewage.
- **Activated sludge process:** It is another method and made by "aeration chamber" sewage from primary sedimentation tank sent into aeration chamber. Where it is mixed with activated sludge, which contains plenty of aerobic bacteria. This process continues for 6 hours and aerobic bacteria oxidize organic matter.
- **Final sedimentation:** Oxidized sewage is now sent into final sedimentation tank and detained for 2½ hrs. The sludge collected is called activated sludge, part of activated sludge, pumped back into aeration chamber and rest into sludge digestion in tank for further treatment.
- **Disposal of effluent:** Finally the water chlorinated and disposed off on land for agriculture.
- **Sludge digestion:** Sludge collected from sludge digestion tank is removed time to time and used as manure.

25. List down waterborne diseases.

BIOLOGICAL (WATERBORNE DISEASES)

- Viral : Viral hepatitis A, Hepatitis E, Poliomyelitis, diarrhea in infants.
- Bacterial : Typhoid fever paratyphoid fever, bacillary, dysentery, *E. coli* diarrhea, cholera

- Protozoal : Amoebiasis, Giardiasis
- Helminthic : Roundworm, threadworm, hydatid disease
- Leptospiral : Weil's disease

THESE DUE TO AQUATIC HOST

- Snail Schistosomiasis
- Cyclops guinea worm, fish, tapeworm
- Chemical dental caries, cyanosis in infant, cardiovascular disease, trachoma, scabies, conjunctivitis
- By insects which breeding into water:
  - Malaria
  - Filaria
  - Kala-azar.

26. Why is there need to control population?

Ans. The population explosion has effects on economic development of the country and living standards of the people. It is a need to control the explosion of population to improve these conditions.

FOR IMPROVEMENT OF ECONOMIC CONDITION

It is big problem of large population, that vacancies are limited and number of candidates are large, which create problem of unemployment, poverty crime and corruption. To control these problems, it is essential to control the population.

FOR SOCIAL CONDITIONS

There are many social problems like begging, smuggling and delinquency which are due to population explosion. These problems affect the social structure. Control on population may help in improving the social conditions.

FOR IMPROVEMENT OF HEALTH CONDITIONS

One of the major reasons for poor health in India and some other developing countries is large size of population, many other problems such as slum area, transportation problem, air, water pollution, communicable diseases occur due to population problem because health services do not reach to all people.

If we want to overcome these problems, we need to control population by adopting different methods.

27. What are the uses of vital statistics?

VITAL STATISTICS

- To measure the state of health of a community and to identify health problems and health needs.
- For comparing the health status of a country with that of another.
- For comparing the present status with that of the past.
- For planning and health administration.
- For evaluation of the progress, success or failure of health program and services in operation.
- For research into community health problems.

28. What are the qualities of community health nurse?

QUALITIES OF COMMUNITY HEALTH NURSE

- Love and coordination with people.
- She should be honest and loyal.
- She should be disciplined and obedient.
- She should be alert and intelligent in observation.
- She should have technical competence.
- She should be dependable and adjustable.
- She should have ability to inspire confidence.
- She should be economical of time, material and energy.
- Should have courtesy and dignity.
- She should be sympathetic and empathetic.
- Intelligent and have common sense.
- Should have patient and sense of humor.
- Should have good physical and mental health.
- Generosity.
- Gentleness and quietness.
- She should possess the required knowledge about legal aspects of nursing.
- She should be able to teach practical nurses and auxiliary workers.
- She should understand and appreciate the importance of good health.
- She should be capable of taking part in the promotion of health and prevention of disease.

29. What are the causes of poor health?

CAUSES OF POOR HEALTH

Poor health is major problem in many developing countries including India. The causes of poor health are:

Environmental Causes

- Lack of safe drinking water
- Lack of basic sanitation
- Crowded, insanitary living conditions
- Pollution of water, food, soil and air.

Socioeconomic Causes

- Poverty
- Illiteracy
- Ignorance
- Customs, traditions, belief and cultural pattern
- Inadequate nutrition
- Lack of personal hygiene
- Rapid population growth.

Other

- Uneven development of health care services and nursing care
- Inadequate primary health care.

30. What are the advantages of small family norms?

ADVANTAGES OF SMALL FAMILY NORMS

- The mother: The mother gets more time to participate in other activities such as education, vocational training and community projects, etc.
- The child: The child will get good atmosphere for his proper physical and psychological growth and development.
- The father: The father can provide children with better education, comfort, food, clothing, and recreation, etc.
- The community: Small family norms help to have enough schools, hospitals and other basic services.

31. What is the immunity?

DEFINITION

It is the ability of the body to recognize, destroy, and eliminate antigenic material.

CLASSIFICATION

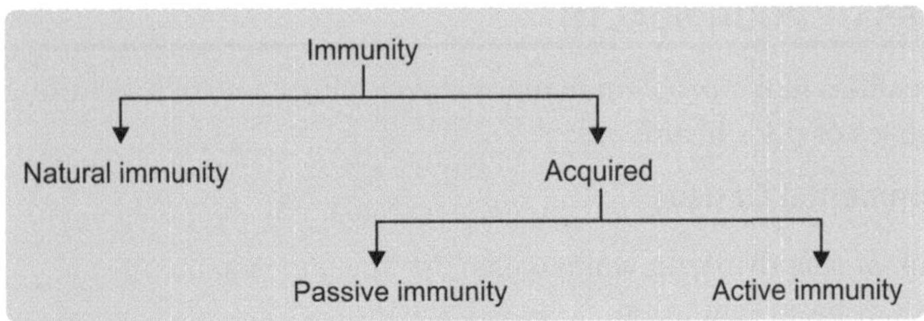

Natural Immunity

It is inherited immunity which individual possesses by genetic make-up. It means, from parents by birth.

Acquired Immunity

It is of two types:

1. Active immunity
2. Passive immunity

Active Immunity

It is an immunity, which develops as a result of infection by pathogenic organism; the body produces own antibody to fight the infection.

Passive Immunity

When antibodies are produced in one person, and are transferred to another to give protection against disease, it is called passive immunity.

32. What are the community health nursing processes?

DEFINITION

Nursing process is a systematic method of collecting data and formulating a nursing care plan in order to provide the most appropriate nursing intervention.

Steps in Nursing Process

- **Recognition:** This process is started by identification of a need. This is based on nursing observation, perception and judgement.
- **Planning:** After assessment of recognition of health need, possible course of action is made. The nurse must decide what action should be taken and whether she is capable of taking such action.

- **Intervention:** In this step, the nurse carries out activities, which decide upon fulfilling the needs of the people. It includes procedures and practices, which are performed by nurses.
- **Evaluation:** In this step, the nurse knows the effectiveness of nursing intervention. It demands a similar range of perception and judgment skill as assessment phase.

33. What are the high-risk families?

HIGH-RISK FAMILIES

These days most important approach developed and promoted by WHO, is to identify the risk group and high-risk families in population. The high risk families are:

Biological Situation

It includes infants, toddler, elderly, female in reproduction age period, pregnant women with high blood pressure, obesity, etc.

Physical Situation

- Rural, slums, etc.
- Living condition, overcrowding.
- Environment: Water supply, unhygienic conditions, over population, over pollution, etc.

Socioeconomic and Cultural Situation

- Social class
- Family disturbance
- Customs, habits and behavior.

In order to reduce the number of high-risk families, primary prevention plays an important role.

These days focus on primary education to the children, early detection of disease, and treatment is given.

34. What are the preventive measures of trachoma in school children?

PREVENTIVE MEASURES OF TRACHOMA

Trachoma is a form of conjunctivitis. It is common in school-going children. Preventive measures are:

Early Diagnosis and Treatment

It is first preventive step in every disease. Daily inspection of children helps in early diagnosis of case and if it is found early, it is treated.

Health Education

Health education to the children about importance of handwashing, using of clean towel, linen, fly control and preventing flies sitting on the feces, attention to good personal hygiene also help in prevention of trachoma.

35. What are the conditions permitting abortion under MTP Act 1971?

Ans. MTP Act came into force in April, 1920. There are five conditions:

- **Medical:** Where the pregnancy is dangerous for mother's health.
- **Eugenic:** Where the risk of the child being born with serious handicapped condition due to physical and mental abnormalities.
- **Humanitarian:** Where pregnancy is as the result of rape.
- **Socioeconomic:** Where the socioeconomic condition is not good for mother and child health.
- **Failure of contraceptive device:** Where the pregnancy is unwanted, due to failure of contraceptive devices.

SOME IMPORTANT QUESTION AND ANSWER RELATED TO NUTRITION

1. (a) Define nutrition
(b) Functions of food
(c) Household methods of food preserving

DEFINE NUTRITION

Nutrition may be defined as the science of food and its relationship to health.

FUNCTIONS OF FOOD

- Provision of energy
- Body building and repair
- Maintenance and regulation of tissue functions.

HOUSEHOLD METHODS OF FOOD PRESERVATION

- **Cold storage:** The home refrigerator has now made it possible to store and preserve a variety of foods. Fruits, vegetables, meads, butter are stored.

- **Drying and dehydration:** Drying removes water, and in the absence of water, microorganisms cannot grow. Fruits, fish, meat preserved by dehydration.
- **Smoking:** Smoke contains phenols, it is used to preserve meat.
- **Salting and pickling:** By adding some spices and condiments along with salt, some foods such as mangoes, meat, fish vegetables may be preserved.
- **Canning:** It is less used because it can not be done properly at home.

2. Sources and effects of vitamin A.

SOURCES

- Liver oil is rich source
- Liver, egg yolk, butter, milk, fish are good sources
- Dark green leafy vegetables such spinach, cabbage, coriander, etc.

Effects of Vitamin 'A'

- **Nightblindness:** Inability to see in dim light is earliest symptom of vitamin A deficiency.
- **Xerophthalmia:** Means dryness of the eye. The white portion of eye becomes dry when the eyelids are kept open for half a minute or so.
- **Bitot's spots:** These are brownish, triangular, raised, foamy patches seen on white portion of the eye.
- **Keratomalacia:** The black portion of eyes become soft and loses its transparency. If it is not treated, it leads to blindness.

3. Methods of cooking.

METHODS OF COOKING

Boiling

Cooking in water at 100°C is called boiling. Rice, roots, pulses, tubers are cooked in this way.

Simmering

Cooking below boiling point at 84°C is called simmering. Meat and fish cooked by simmering.

Steaming

Pressure cooking is better for steaming. It also save fuel and time.

Stewing

In stewing, 80°C temperature is applied and the food is half covered with liquid. Nutrients not lost. It is used for meat cooking.

Frying

This is of two types—In shallow and deep. Shallow frying is suitable for eggs, dosa, etc. In deep frying you need more hot oil to immerse the food for cooking pakora, puri, cutlets, etc.

Roasting

Food is directly exposed to heat or flame it is called roasting. Chicken and mutton cooked in this way.

Baking

Cooking by dry heat in oven is called baking. It is expensive and slow method.

Broiling and Grilling

It is cooking by direct dry heat. It can be done, either in a grill or heavy pan or direct on flame kabab, cheese, brinjals are cooked by this method.

4. Disadvantages of milk boiling.

DISADVANTAGES OF MILK BOILING

- Boiling kills all organisms present in the milk, including the useful lactic acid bacteria.
- It destroys vitamin C and vitamin B mostly.
- Proteins in the milk are coagulated.
- Boiling gives a cooked taste to the milk due to burning.
- The enzymes are destroyed.

5. Functions of protein.

FUNCTIONS OF PROTEIN

- Proteins help in synthesis of enzymes immunoglobulin, plasma proteins and hormones.
- Proteins help in growth and repair of body tissues.
- Proteins are secondary sources of energy during deficiency of carbohydrates and fats. It provides 4 kilo calories of energy.

- Proteins supply the material for building of cells.
- Proteins are chief sole matter of muscles, organs or endocrine glands.
- They are also the component of skin, nails, hair, blood cells, serum and teeth.
- Except bile and urine, all of body fluids contain protein.
- They are important for body regulation.

6. Nutrients deficiency disease.

Ans.

Nutrients	Deficiency
1. Protein, fat, carbohydrates	Protein energy malnutrition: • Kwashiorkor • Marasmus
2. Vitamin A	• Night blindness
	• Xerophthalmia • Bitots spots • Keratomalacia
3. Vitamin D	• Rickets in children
	• Osteomalacia in adults
4. Vitamin B	• Beriberi, encephalopathy
5. Nicotine	• Pellagra, dermatitis, underweight diarrhea, dementia
6. Iron, folic acid	• Anemia
7. Vitamin C	• Scurvy, lack of appetite, weakness, bleeding of gums
8. Iodine	• Goiter
9. Calcium	• Weak bones and teeth
10. Fluorine	• Dental caries
11. Vitamin E	• Poor skin integrity

7. Water and fat soluble vitamins.

WATER AND FAT SOLUBLE VITAMINS

1. **Fat soluble vitamins:**
   Vit A Vit D Vit E Vit K
2. **Water soluble vitamins:**
   - Thiamine (vit B1)
   - Riboflavin (vit B2)
   - Nicotinic acid
   - Pyridoxine (vit B6)
   - Pantothenic acid

- Vit B12
- Folic acid
- Ascorbic acid (vit C)

8. **Source of All Nutrients**

Ans.

S. No.	Nutrient	Source
1.	Protein	**Animal** – Milk, egg, meat, fist **Plant** – Pulses, cereals, nuts
2.	Fat	**Animal:** Ghee, butter, fat of meat, fish oil
3.	Carbohydrate	**Rice, wheat, root, tubers; Animal:** Butter, ghee, egg, Milk, liver, fish
4.	Vit A	**Vegetables:** Green leafy vegetables, spinach, amaranth corian-der, drum stick leaves, mangoes, papaya, tomatoes, fish liver oils.
5.	Vit D	Sunlight
6.	Vit E	**Food:** Egg, yolk, liver, fish, fish oil
7.	Vit 'K'	It is available in meats, fruits and vegetables, oils of sunflower seeds, cotton.
8.	Thiamine	Fresh green leafy vegetables, fruits
9.	Riboflavin	In unmilled cereals, pulses and groundnuts
10.	Niacin	Milk and milk products, eggs, liver, green leafy veg
11.	Folic acid	Grain cereals, pulses, nuts, meat, liver and chicken.
12.	Vit B12	Green leaves, pulses, nuts, whole grain liver, fish, egg, milk
13.	Vit 'C'	Amla, gooseberry, guavas; green leafy vegetables, meat and milk.
14.	Minerals	In all foods
15.	Calcium	Milk, egg, meat, green, leafy vegetables, fruits
16.	Iron	Liver, kidney, meat, egg yolk, cereals, pulses, green vegetables
17.	Iodine	Sea, water, and sea food
18.	Flourine	Drinking water.

9. **Difference between normal diet and therapeutic.**

Ans.

Therapeutic diet	Normal diet
• It is planed according to the need of patients and according to disease condition	• It includes carbohydrate, proteins, fat, vitamins, minerals in adequate amount as needed by body to maintain good health status
• It includes generally soft and liquid diet	

10. Describe the factors contributing towards good health.

Ans. There are so many factors that contribute towards good health:

PROPER NUTRITION

Adequate nutrition is essential for good health. More attention is given on vulnerable groups such as infants, children, pregnant and lactating women and nutritional needs of the elderly must be met.

HEALTHY ENVIRONMENT

A healthy environment contributes in good health and well-being of individuals and communities. Poor environment is major cause of ill health in many developing countries.

GOOD HEATH HABITS

Good health habits such as:

- Exercise
- No smoking
- No drug abuse
- Eating healthy diet, avoiding spices and fast food.

People must assume responsibility for their own health by adopting good habits.

EARLY DIAGNOSIS AND TREATMENT

Early diagnosis of disease helps to prevents the health problems and early treatment prevents complications:

HEALTH EDUCATION

Health education to people about health also contributes in maintaining good health. In education activities include following topics:

- Education about personal hygiene
- Education about adopting healthy life-style
- Education about diet
- For prevention of illness.

SOCIOECONOMIC FACTORS

Good income in family also helps in good health. Per capita income related to health of family members.

FAMILY SIZE, BIRTH RATE

Increased, size of family related with the health of family. If the family size is small all the basic needs are completed.

HEALTH EXAMINATION, SCREENING AND IMMUNIZATION

These all factors also contribute in good health. Immunization against infectious diseases prevents ill health.

RECORDS

- It is important to keep record of all health events.
- These are the factors contributing towards health.

11. Principles of cooking.

Ans. Cooking is an art, which changes the flavor, texture, appearance and taste of food and makes it easily digestible. The basic principles are:

- Food must not be over-cooked or under-cooked to prevent the loss of essential nutrients.
- It sterilizes food by killing microorganisms, parasitic ova and eggs.
- There should be variety in cooking. It makes many dishes without destroying nutrients.
- Excessive use of condiments likes salt and red pepper may lead to common problems like hypertension, piles, etc.
- Good cooking increases the acceptability of food.
- If must be done in a hygienic place. Handling and storing of food must also be done in some hygienic place.
- Cooking area must have a sufficient distance from sanitary area.

12. Principles of recording and reporting.

Ans. Records are written legal documents. Following principles are kept in mind while writing records:

- It should be written clearly, accurately, appropriately and legibly.
- All entries should be signed by the individual who writes them.
- Records should be written correct. Any errors on the records should be avoided.
- Records should be written in chronological order according to date and time.
- Use only standard abbreviations which are known by all health workers.
- Records should be truthful, brief and complete.

- Recording and reporting should be done immediately after an observation and event.
- Records should be kept confidential.
- It should not be discussed with strange persons.
- Records should not be handed over to any person without permission.

13. Effects of noise and air pollution.

EFFECTS OF NOISE

Noise a effects on ears. It causes deafness, which may become permanent if the noise exposure is too high:

- Hearing loss
- Disturbance in communication
- Noise interferes with speech
- Inability to concentrate
- Loss of speech or disturbance to sleep
- Noise creates accident in industries
- Physiological changes in the body such as rise in blood pressure.

EFFECTS OF AIR POLLUTION

Health effects of air pollution are of two types immediate and delayed.

- **Immediate:** Immediate effect are acute bronchitis or even immediate death by suffocation.
- **Delayed:** These effects include chronic bronchitis, lung cancer, asthma, emphysema, respiratory allergies, etc.

14. Role of nurse in family welfare.

ROLE OF A NURSE IN FAMILY WELFARE

Administrative Role

She participates in the organization of family welfare program at national or community level.

Supervisory Role

She is responsible in supervision of health workers such as Auxiliary nurse, Midwife (ANM), New staff, students, etc. She help the staff in providing health services.

Functional Role

The primary function of nurse in family planning is finding eligible couples and making referral to adopt suitable family planning methods.

Educational Role

She educates the family and community about family life, family planning, methods of regulating fertility, etc.

Role in Research

She participates in research activities related to family welfare program.

Role in Evaluation

Evaluation is an important part of planning for nursing services.

Community Health Nursing
November 2016

Time: 3 Hours **Maximum Marks: 75**

Note: *Attempt all questions in continuity:*

1. **(a) Define the following terms:**
   i. Communication
   ii. IMR
   iii. Eradication
   iv. Health education
   v. WHO

   (b) Write the purposes of home visiting.
   (c) Write the principles of Primary Health Care. **(5 + 5 + 5 = 15)**

2. **(a) Write the causes of poor health in India.**
   (b) Write the signs and symptoms of measles.
   (c) Write the prevention and control of communicable diseases.
   (5 + 5 + 5 = 15)

3. **(a) What are the principles of Health Education?**
   (b) What are the components of School Health Services?
   (c) Explain the functions of female health worker. **(5 + 5 + 5 = 15)**

4. **(a) Explain the indicators of Health.**
   (b) Discuss the methods of Family Planning.
   (c) Discuss Records and Reports. **(5 + 5 + 5 = 15)**

5. **Write short notes on the following:**
   (a) Tuberculosis or enlist the minor ailments
   (b) Dimensions of health
   (c) Immunity or MTP **(5 + 5 + 5 = 15)**

SOLVED QUESTION PAPER NOVEMBER 2016

1. **(a) Define the following terms:**
    i. Communication
    ii. IMR
    iii. Eradication
    iv. Health Education
    v. WHO

    (b) Write the purposes of home visiting.

    (c) Write the principles of Primary Health Care.

COMMUNICATION

It is process of exchanging or shaping ideas, feelings and information.

IMR

Infant mortality rate is the ratio of deaths under 1 year of age in a given year to the total number of live births in the same year, usually expressed as a rate per 1000 live births.

ERADICATION

Termination of all transmission of infection by extermination of the infectious agent through surveillance and containment.

HEALTH EDUCATION

The process by which individuals and groups of people learn to behave in a manner conducive to the promotion, maintenance or restoration of health.

WHO

It is specialized, nonpolitical health agency of the united nations with headquarters at Geneva.

PURPOSE OF HOME VISITING

Refer paper 2010 question no 3(a)

PRINCIPLES OF PRIMARY HEALTH CARE

Refer paper 2010 question no 5(a)

2. **(a) Write the causes of poor health in India.**

    (b) Write the signs and symptoms of measles.

    (c) Write the prevention and control of communicable diseases.

CAUSES OF POOR HEALTH IN INDIA

Refer important theory question no 29

SIGNS AND SYMPTOMS OF MEASLES

Prodromal Stage

It begins 10 days after infection and lasts until day 14. It is characterized by fever, sneezing and nasal discharge, cough, redness of eyes, lacrimation and photophobia. A day or two before the appearance of the Koplik's spots.

Eruptive Stage

This phase is characterized by a typical, dusty-red, macular or maculo-popular rash, which begins behind the ears and spreads rapidly in a few hour over the face and neck and extend down to the body.

Post Measles Stage

The child will have lost weight and will remain weak for a number of days.

PREVENTION AND CONTROL OF COMMUNICABLE DISEASES

Nurses play a vital role in prevention and eradication of communicable disease. Here are measures to control:

Early Diagnosis

Nurses make early diagnosis while by confirming with laboratory methods.

Notification

Notification is done by health worker within 24 hour of occurrence of case to the primary health center. Purpose of notification is to enable further action to be taken to control the spread of infection.

Isolation

Nurses isolate the patient suffering from disease, i.e. communicable.

Treatment

Nurse provides treatment or enable patient to get treatment. It is an important aspect of the control of an infectious disease.

Surveillance

It is a new concept in disease control. Nurses do house to house visiting.

Disinfection

In this, nurse has to educate people regarding disinfection.

Blocking the Channels of Transmission

Nurses has to educate people regarding measures to control communicable disease. These are:

- Disinfection of water supplies
- Safe disposal of human excrete and solid waste
- Control of insects and rodents
- Improving the standard of food hygiene, etc.

Protecting the Susceptible Population

It is the nurse's prime responsibility to educate the community people regarding prevention and treatment of communicable diseases.

Immunization

Key to the prevention of many infections diseases lie in immunization. It is an important weapon in control of spread of infection.

Health Education

Successful control of any communicable disease requires community participation and proper health education.

Proper Treatment

Proper treatment with adequate doses of medicine for diagnosed cases.

3. (a) What are the principles of Health Education?
(b) What are the components of School Health Services?
(c) Explain the functions of female health worker.

PRINCIPLES OF HEALTH EDUCATION

Refer important theory question no 6.

COMPONENTS OF SCHOOL HEALTH SERVICES

Refer important theory question no 22.

FUNCTIONS OF FEMALE HEALTH WORKER

Refer paper 2010 question no 5(b)

4. (a) Explain the indicators of Health.
(b) Discuss the methods of Family Planning.
(c) Discuss Records and Reports.

INDICATORS OF HEALTH

Refer paper 2010 question no 6(c)

METHODS OF FAMILY PLANNING

Refer paper 2004 question no 4(a)

RECORDS AND REPORTS

Refer important theory question no 12

5. **Write short notes on the following:**
   (a) Tuberculosis or enlist the minor ailments
   (b) Dimensions of health
   (c) Immunity or MTP

TUBERCULOSIS

It is infectious disease caused by *Mycobacterium tuberculosis.*

Source of Infection

- Infected person
- Sputum and saliva of infected person
- Articles contaminated by the infected person
- By coughing, sneezing.

Incubation Period

3 to 6 weeks

Signs and Symptoms

- Persistent cough of about 3 to 4 weeks duration
- Continuous fever
- Chest pain
- Hemoptysis

Control of Tuberculosis

The control measures consist of a curative and preventive component.

Health Education

Health education should be given to the people regarding its spreading and controlling because it is useful tool for prevention of tuberculosis.

Early Identification and Prompt Treatment

Detect signs and symptoms early, identify the cases and notify the health for prompt treatment.

Chemotherapy

Chemotherapy is indicated in every case of active tuberculosis.

Drugs used for treatment is:
- Rifampicin (RMP)
- INH
- Streptomycin
- Pyrazinamide
- Ethambutol

DOTS

Today new strategy introduce for to ensure cure by providing the most effective medicine and confirming that it is taken. In DOTS during the intensive phase of treatment a health worker or other trained person watches as the patient swallows the drug in his presence.

MINOR AILMENTS

A minor ailment is a less serious medical condition that does not require lab or blood tests, e.g.
- Cold sores
- Mild eczema
- Oral thrush
- Heartburn
- Hay fever
- Nasal congestion
- Skin rash
- Fungal skin infection
- Yeast infections
- Cough
- Cold
- Minor cuts

Treatment and Prevention of Minor Ailments

Assessment

Take history and quick physical examination, find the cause, make the diagnosis and plan for care provided treatment and nursing care in a comprehensive manner.

Evaluating the care and condition of the patient.

Principles of Managing Minor Ailments

- Ensure a safe and healthful environment for a patient
- Treat the risk to prevent any possible complication
- Use the opportunities of healthful environment during care
- Keep continuous watch over the patient's condition and vital signs during the entire period of care
- Always remember the limitation in providing Rx or follow the physician
- Help the members in coping with situation and prepare them for taking care of sick at home
- Respect the belief of patients.

DIMENSIONS OF HEALTH

Physical Dimension

The state of physical health implies the notion of perfect functioning of the body. The signs and symptoms of physical health are a good complexion, a clean skin, bright eyes, lustrous hair, not too fat, a sweet breath , a good appetite, sound sleep, regular bowels and bladder movement, coordinated bodily movements.

Evaluation of Physical Health

- Self-assessment of overall health
- Inquiry into symptoms of ill health and risk factors
- Inquiry into medications
- Inquiry into level of activity
- Inquiry into use of medical services
- Standardized questionnaires for cardiovascular diseases
- Clinical examination
- Nutrition and dietary assessment

Mental Dimension

Mental health is not mere absence of mental illness. Good mental health is the ability to respond to the many varied experiences of life with flexibility and a sense of purpose. It is a state of balance between individual and the surrounding world.

Characteristic of Mentally Healthy Person

- A mentally healthy person free from internal conflicts
- He is well adjusted with others
- He searches for identity
- He has a strong sense of self-esteem
- He knows himself, his needs, problems and goals
- He has good self-control, balances, rationality and emotionality
- He faces problems and tries to solve them.

Assessment

- Mental status questionnaires
- Interviewers

Social Dimension

Social well-being implies harmony and integration within the individual between each individual and other members of society and between individuals and the world in which they live.

The social dimension of health includes the levels of social skills one possess, social functioning and the ability to see oneself as a member of a larger society.

Spiritual Diversion

Spiritual health in this context refers to that part of the individual which reaches out and strives for meaning and purpose in life. It includes integrity, principles and ethics.

Emotional Dimension

Mental and emotional dimension have been seen as one element or as two closely related elements. Mental health can be seen as knowing or cognition while emotional health relates to feeling.

Vocational Dimension

It is new dimension when work is fully adapted to human goals, capacities and limitations, work often plays a role in promoting both physical and mental health. It helps to improve physical capacity, achievement and self- realization.

Others:

- Philosophical dimension
- Cultural dimension
- Socioeconomic dimension
- Environmental dimension
- Educational dimension
- Nutritional dimension
- Curative dimension
- Preventive dimension

IMMUNITY

Refer important theory question no 32

MTP

Refer important theory question no 35

Community Health Nursing
October 2015

Time: 3 Hours | **Maximum Marks: 75**

Note: *Attempt all questions. Please attempt all parts of the question in sequence.*

1. Define the following: 1×10 = 10

(a) Epidemiology (b) Malnutrition
(c) Family (d) Epidemic
(e) Primary Health Care (f) Health
(g) Immunity (h) Nutrition
(i) PEM (j) Balance Diet

2. (a) Define the Community Health Nursing. 2+5+8 = 15

(b) Write down the principles of Community Health Nursing.

(c) Write about the functions of Community Health Nurse.

3. (a) Define Home Visiting. 2+5+8 = 15

(b) Write down the purpose of Home Visiting.

(c) Write about the functions of Community Health Nurse.

4. (a) Define Health Education. 2+5+8 = 15

(b) Write the principles of Health Education.

(c) Explain immunization schedule.

5. Write short notes on any four of the following: 5×4 = 20

(a) Bag Technique (b) Water Pollution
(c) Referral System (d) Standing Order/Instructions
(e) WHO

SOLVED QUESTION PAPER 2015

1. Define the followings:

(a) Epidemiology (b) Malnutrition
(c) Family (d) Epidemic
(e) Primary Health Care (f) Health
(g) Immunity (h) Nutrition
(i) PEM (j) Balance Diet

EPIDEMIOLOGY

Epidemiology is concerned with the pattern of disease occurrence in human population and of the factors that influence there patterns.

MALNUTRITION

It is a condition, which occurs when the body does not get the proper kind of food in the amounts needed for maintaining health.

FAMILY

It is defined as 'a group of individuals they have blood relation, living together and eating from a common kitchen, living under one roof'.

EPIDEMIC

Epidemic means an outbreak of disease in a community in excess of normal expectation derived from common source.

PRIMARY HEALTH CARE

PHC is essential for health care made universally accessible to individuals and acceptable to them, through their full participation and at a cost that the community and country can afford.

HEALTH

According to WHO 'Health' is a state of complete physical, mental, social well-being and not merely an absence of disease or infirmity.

IMMUNITY

It is the power of body to fight against infection.

NUTRITION

Nutrition may be defined as the science of food and its relationship to health.

PEM

Protein Energy Malnutrition, when protein and calories not enough in diet that cause PEM. It mainly occurs in childrens.

BALANCED DIET

Balanced diet is the one which consists of all the required nutrients in correct or adequate amount for proper maintainance and regulation of body functions.

2. (a) Define the Community Health Nursing.
(b) Write down the principles of Community Health Nursing.
(c) Write about the functions of Community Health Nurse.

Ans. *Refer last year question papers.*

3. (a) Define Home Visiting.
(b) Write down the purpose of Home Visiting.
(c) Write about the principles of Home Visiting.

HOME VISITING

It is a technique through which nurse or health team go to door step (home to home) to assess the health status of people and give necessary care to sick people.

PURPOSE OF HOME VISITING

Refer paper 2010 question no 3 (a)

PRINCIPLES OF HOME VISITING

Refer paper October 2006 question no 4 (c)

4. (a) Define Health Education.
(b) Write the principles of Health Education.
(c) Explain immunization schedule.

DEFINE HEALTH EDUCATION

Refer Paper September 2005 question no 4 (a)

PRINCIPLES OF HEALTH EDUCATION

Refer Paper September 2005 question no 4 (b)

IMMUNIZATION SCHEDULE

Refer paper 2004 question no 5 (b)

5. Write short notes on any four of the followings:

(a) Bag Technique
(b) Water Pollution
(c) Referral System
(d) Standing Order/Instructions
(e) WHO

BAG TECHNIQUE

Refer paper September 2005 question no 5 (b)

WATER POLLUTION

Refer paper October 2007 question no 6 (4)

REFERRAL SYSTEM

Refer paper September 2005 question no 6 (c)

STANDING ORDER

Standing orders are specific instruction regarding any treatment for conditions that nurse and other health workers may meet in homes, schools and in industries while a doctor is not readily available.

Classification of Minor Ailments

1. Fever
2. Sore throat
3. Cough
4. Inflamed eyes
5. Burns
6. Toothache
7. Earache
8. diarrhea
9. Skin rashes
10. Animal bite
11. Snake bite
12. Fracture
13. Heat stroke
14. Anemia
15. Epistaxis
16. Shock
17. Scabies
18. Fits
19. Constipation

Responsibility of Nurse and Other Health Worker

- Obtain information from family and patient in initiate nursing care
- Be sure what has been done
- Record vital signs and urine examination
- Identify the problem and needs of the individuals
- Implement nursing care following standing instructions

- Reassure family and patient
- Explain disease, causation, prevention, complication, etc.
- Evaluate the progress
- Notify if any communicable disease is suspected.

WHO (WORLD HEALTH ORGANIZATION)

The WHO is a specialized non political health agency of the United Nations with headquarters at Geneva.

Objective: The objective of the WHO is 'the attainment by all peoples of the highest level of health'.

The current objective of WHO is the attainment by all people of the world by the year 2000 AD of a level of health that will permit them to lead a socially and economically productive life also known as Health for All by 2000 AD.

Membership: Membership in WHO is open to all countries while most countries are members of both the UN and of WHO, there are some differences. In 1948 the WHO had 56 members. In 1996 WHO had 190 member states and two associate members.

Work of WHO

- Prevention and control of specific diseases
- Development of comprehensive health services
- Family health
- Environmental health
- Health statistics
- Biomedical research
- Health literature and information
- Co-operation with other organization

Community Health Nursing
September 2015

Time: 3 Hours **Maximum Marks: 75**

Note: *Attempt all questions, attempt all parts of question in continuity.*

1. a. **Describe the functions of protein.** 5+5+5 = 15
   b. **Write about principles of primary healthcare.**
   c. **What is the role of community health nurse in primary healthcare.**
2. a. **Write about the concept of health and disease.** 7+8 = 15
   b. **Explain about different health problems in India.**
3. **Explain the following:** 5+5+5 = 15
   a. Air pollution
   b. Functions of under five clinics
   c. WHO
4. a. **Explain healthcare delivery system.** 5+10 = 15
   b. **Write about healthcare delivery system at village level.**
5. **Write short notes on any three of the following:** 5+5+5 = 15
   a. Home visiting
   b. Measles
   c. PHC
   d. Immunization
   e. AIDS

SOLVED QUESTION PAPER SEPTEMBER 2015

1. a. **Describe the functions of protein.**
   b. **Write about principles of primary healthcare.**
   c. **What is the role of community health nurse in primary healthcare?**

FUNCTIONS OF PROTEIN

Refer paper 2009 Q no 4 (b) functions of protein

PRINCIPLES OF PRIMARY HEALTHCARE

Refer paper 2009 Q no 3(b)

ROLE OF COMMUNITY HEALTH NURSE IN PHC

Refer paper 2009 Q no 3(c)

2. a. Write about the concept of health and disease.
b. Explain about different health problems in India.

CONCEPT OF HEALTH AND DISEASE

Heath: A state of complete physical, mental and social well-being of an individual and not merely an absence of disease or infirmity.

As per the definition, health is three dimensional—the physical, the mental and the social.

Disease: A condition, in which body health is impaired and performance of vital functions in the body is interrupted. In other words deslase is a physiological or psychological dysfunction of the body.

HEALTH PROBLEMS IN INDIA

Every country has its own health problem depending upon the standard of living of its people, size of population, the health problems of India may be classified as below:

- Communicable disease problems
- Nutritional problems
- Environmental sanitation problems
- Medical care problems
- Population problems.

Communicable Disease Problem

Communicable decease continue to be a major problem in India, whereas they have been largely controlled in the developed countries such as USA and UK. It has been estimated that nearly 54 percent of deaths in India are due to communicable diseases.

- Malaria
- Tuberculosis
- Diarrheal diseases
- Acute respiratory infections
- Leprosy
- Filarial
- STD

- AIDS
- Others.

Nutritional Problems

Malnutrition is widely prevalence in India. The specific nutritional problems are:

- Protein-calorie-malnutrition
- Endemic goiter
- Vitamins deficiency disorders
- Anemias
- Lathyrism
- Fluorosis.

Environmental Sanitation Problems

Lack of safe water supply and sanitary methods for excreta disposal are the chief problems. Surveys indicate that about 85% of people in rural areas defecate in open fields and cause soil pollutions. During 2008, safe water was available to 96% of the urban and 84% of rural population. Adequate facilities for excreta disposal were available only to 54% of the urban and hardly 21% of the rural population.

Medical Care Problems

Medical care in India is mostly based on western medicine. Modern medical care has indeed become costly and complex. The current criticism is that medical care in India is mostly urban oriented, curative in nature and not accessible to the bulk of the rural population. Approximately 80% of health facilities are concentrated in urban areas. Even in urban areas, there is an uneven distribution of doctors. Thus the major medical care problems are inequitable distribution of health resources between rural and urban areas.

Population Problems

The population problem is the biggest problem facing the county. The 2011 census showed a population of 1.21 billion and the current growth rate of 1.64%. The population explosion has affected economic. Development of the country and the living standards of the people.

3. Explain the following:

a. Air pollution
b. Functions of under five clinics
c. WHO

AIR POLLUTION

Refer paper 2008 Q no 2.

FUNCTIONS OF UNDER FIVE CLINICS

Refer paper 2007 Q no 4(b).

WORLD HEALTH ORGANIZATION (WHO)

World health organization was established in the April 1948. The headquarter of WHO is situated at Geneva.

Objectives

- It defines health as a, 'state of complete physical, mental and social well-being and not merely the absence of disease or infirmity'.
- It declares that the attainment of highest level of health is one of the fundamental rights of every human being without destination of race, religion, political belief, economic and social condition.
- It recognizes that the health of all people is fundamental to the attainment of peace and security and to the abolition of wars.
- It fixes the responsibility on the government of the countries to provide adequate health and social welfare measures for the benefit of their citizens.
- It affirms that the health of one country is of benefit to all other countries.
- It also suggests that health education of all the people is essential to fullest attainment of health.

Membership

Membership is open to all the countries. The countries which do not maintain the international relations are admitted as associate members. During 1948, WHO had 56 members, by 1996 WHO had 190 members, state and two associate members.

Functions

- Health services
- Health information and literature
- Health research

4. a. Explain healthcare delivery system.
b. Write about healthcare delivery system at village level.

HEALTHCARE DELIVERY SYSTEM

The healthcare services in India are organized at three levels, each level supported by the higher level, to which the patient is referred.

1. Primary healthcare
2. Secondary healthcare
3. Tertiary level of healthcare.

Primary Healthcare

It is the first level of contract between the individual/family and the health system, where basic, essential services are provided at this level, the health services are provided even at the individual's door level, i.e. at the grass-root level. In India, this care is provided by primary health centers, subcenters, supplemented by the services of the village health guides, the Anganwadi workers and trained Dais.

Secondary Level of Healthcare

At this level, halt the progress of disease. Thus essentially curative services are provided in taluka hospitals and community health centers.

Tertiary Level of Healthcare

At this level, services of specialties are made available to the people. This type of care is provided in regional/central/ape institution such as district hospitals, teaching hospitals.

HEALTHCARE DELIVERY SYSTEM AT VILLAGE LEVEL

This is the first level of contact between the health system and the individual/family of the community. At this level, the primary healthcare is provided not by the medical personnel but by the non-medical personnel such as village health guide, dais, and anganwadi worker. They are working under the following schemes respectively:

- Village health guide scheme
- Training of local dais
- ICDS scheme.

Village Health Guide Scheme

This was launched on 2nd October 1977. A village health guide is one who has an aptitude for social service. One village health guide is selected for each village or 1000 rural population.

Selection Guidelines

- She must be a permanent, local resident of that village.
- She must be literate, as to read, write and maintain records.
- She must be acceptable to all section of society.
- She must be willing to do community health work for 2 to 3 hours a day.

Training Time

After selection, she is given training in the primary health center by medical offices for 3 months on the basic aspects of health such as personal hygiene, sanitation, health education, first aid, ORT, family welfare, etc. with the stipend of ₹ 200 per month for training period.

Training of Local Dais (Trained Birth Attendant)

This is another component of rural health scheme, launched in 1978. Traditional birth attendants are the only people who are available in the villages to conduct the deliveries. After training, the traditional birth attendant is called trained birth attendant.

Training

Training is provided in PHC by lady medical officer for 1 month with a stipend of ₹ 300 per month.

During these 30 days, she will have training at PHC for 2 days in a week and remaining 4 days of the week, except Sundays. She will accompany the health worker female to the village during her training, she is required to conduct at least 2 deliveries under the guidance and supervision of HWF or ANM or health assistant female.

After the training, she is given a certificate and a maternity kit.

Anganwadi Workers

Angan means 'courtyard'. Anganwadi worker is a local lady, studied up to 10th standard, selected as a worker for 1000 population to provide basic health services such as MCH. She is the 'key' person to deliver the services under ICDS scheme. She caters the services to a population of 1000, covering about 170 children between 0 to 6 years, 30 expectant mothers, 15 lactating mothers and 200 women in the age group of 15 to 44 years.

Training

She is trained for 4 months in various aspects of health, nutrition and child development after the training, she works as a part time worker and she is paid an honorarium of about ₹ 500 per month.

5. **Write short notes on any three of the following:**
   a. Home visiting
   b. Measles
   c. PHC
   d. Immunization
   e. AIDS

HOME VISITING

Refer paper January 2012 Q no 2

MEASLES

It is caused by paramyxovirus.

Incubation Period

10 to 14 days.

Clinical Features

Features occur in two stages:
1. Prodromal stage
2. Exanthematous stage.

Prodromal Stage

It is also called pre-eruptive stage or catarrhal stage. Characterized by fever anorexia, cough, conjunctival congestion, photophobia, swelling of lower lids, sunny nose, flushing of the face.

One or two days before the appearance of rashes, Koplik's spots appear on the buccal mucous membrane.

Exanthematous Stage (Eruptive Stage)

Rashes appear on 4th day of fever, first behind the ears, then on the forehead, face and down the trunk, slowly taking 2 to 3 days to progress to the hands and lower extremities. Rashes are pink colored and maculepapular. At this age, temperature is very high about 104°F continuity another 1 or 2 days.

From the 5th or 6th day rashes begin to disappear in the same order they had appeared, no permanent pockmark are left behind.

Management and Nursing Care

1. Isolation in a well-ventilated room
2. Concurrent disinfection of nasal and throat secretions
3. TPR chart maintained 4th hourly
4. Light and clean clothes
5. Eyes are washed with sterile normal saline
6. Antipyretics to control fever
7. Prophylactic antibiotics may be given
8. Plenty of water and fruit juice given
9. Watch for the complications
10. Terminal disinfection of the room.

Prevention and Control

This is done by active and passive immunization.
Active immunization: This is done by using live attenuated vaccines.
Measles vaccine of multiple antigen: MMR.

PHC

Refer paper 2004 Q no 3(a)
Refer paper 2009 Q no 3(c)

IMMUNIZATION

Refer paper 2010 Q no 6(a)

AIDS

Acquired immune deficiency syndrome.

Mode of Transmission

(a) By direct sexual contact
(b) By infected blood transfusion
(c) By using infected syringes and needles
(d) By vertical transmission.

Prevention and Control of AIDS

Refer paper 2005 Q no 6(e).

Community Health Nursing
December 2013

Time: 3 Hours **Maximum Marks: 75**

Note: *Attempt all questions. Please attempt parts of the same question altogether and not in parts.*

1. **(a) Explain functions of primary health center.** 5+5+5 = 15
   (b) Explain the principles of primary health care.
   (c) Write down the principles of health education.
2. **(a) Explain the objectives of school health program.** 5+5+5 = 15
   (b) Explain the objective of under five clinics.
   (c) Explain the objectives of community health nursing practice.
3. **(a) Explain different methods of cooking food.** 5+5+5 = 15
   (b) Explain vitamin A deficiency diseases.
   (c) List the water soluble and fat soluble vitamins.
4. **(a) Explain different barriers of communication.** 5+5+5 = 15
   (b) Explain family welfare services.
   (c) Explain characteristics of healthy individual.
5. **Write short notes on any three of the following:** 5+5+5 = 15
   (a) Sterilization
   (b) Tuberculosis
   (c) Measles
   (d) Dengue fever
   (e) Qualities of a community health nurse

SOLVED QUESTION PAPER DECEMBER 2013

1. **(a) Explain functions of primary health center.**
   (b) Explain the principles of primary health care.
   (c) Write down the principles of health education.

FUNCTIONS OF PRIMARY HEALTH CENTER (PHC)

Refer Paper 2004 question no 3 (a)

PRINCIPLES OF PRIMARY HEALTH CENTER (PHC)

Refer Paper 2005 question no 3 (a)

PRINCIPLES OF HEALTH EDUCATION

Refer Paper 2005 question no 4 (b)

2. (a) Explain the objectives of school health program.
(b) Explain the objectives of under five clinics.
(c) Explain the objectives of community health nursing practice.

OBJECTIVES OF SCHOOL HEALTH PROGRAM

Refer Paper 2006 question no 4 (d)

OBJECTIVE OF UNDER FIVE CLINICS

Refer Paper 2004 question no 5 (a)

OBJECTIVES OF COMMUNITY HEALTH NURSING PRACTICE

Refer Paper 2007 question no 3 (a)

3. (a) Explain different methods of cooking food.
(b) Explain vitamin A deficiency diseases.
(c) List the water-soluble and fat-soluble vitamins.

METHODS OF COOKING FOOD

Refer Paper 2004 question no 5 (c)

VITAMIN 'A' DEFICIENCY DISEASES

Refer important theory question no 2 page no 25

WATER-SOLUBLE AND FAT-SOLUBLE VITAMINS

Refer Paper 2006 question no 2 (c)

4. (a) Explain different barriers of communication.
(b) Explain family welfare services.
(c) Explain characteristics of healthy individual.

BARRIERS OF COMMUNICATION

Refer Paper 2008 question no 5 (b)

FAMILY WELFARE SERVICES

Refer Paper 2008 question no 5 (d)

CHARACTERISTICS OF HEALTHY INDIVIDUAL

Refer Paper 2006 question no 3 (c)

5. Write short notes on any three of the following:

(a) Sterilization
(b) Tuberculosis
(c) Measles
(d) Dengue fever
(e) Qualities of a community health nurse

STERILIZATION

Sterilization for men and women is a permanent method for individuals who do not want any more children.

Female Sterilization

There are two common procedures for female sterilization as described below:

- **Laparoscopy:** A laparoscopy is used for sterilization purpose. The abdomen is inflated with carbon dioxide or nitrous oxide and laparoscope is introduced to visualize the fallopian tubes. Then the clips are applied to occlude the tubes. It is not advisable 6 weeks after delivery.
- **Mini lap:** It is a permanent contraception for women who do not want more children. It is safe and simple surgical procedure. A small incision 2.5–3 cm is made in the woman's abdomen and the two fallopian tubes are blocked off or cut.

Male Sterilization

- **Vasectomy:** In this method, the vas deferens, the ejaculatory duct is blocked to prevent the sperms from being released. It is a safe simple and quick surgical procedure which can done in clinic. A small opening in the man's scrotum is made and both tubes of vas deferens are closed off which carry sperm from testicles. A man becomes sterile after about 3 months or when 20 ejaculations has been completed after the procedure. The man is advised to wear T-bandage for 15 days and also not lift heavy object for 15 days.

- **No scalpel vasectomy:** It is a safe minimally invasive procedure that reduces complications occurring in conventional. In India, the technique was introduced in 1992. It has advantages such as no incision and no stitches are required. This reduces the stress and anxiety leading up to the procedure. The procedure is faster as it takes about 10 minutes to complete. Even there are less chances of infection or bleeding and is effective also.

TUBERCULOSIS (TB)

It is a chronic infectious disease caused by tubercle bacilli (*mycobacterium tuberculosis*). The disease affects lungs and causes pulmonary tuberculosis.

Mode of Transmission

- **Droplet infection:** Coughing, talking, sneezing, etc.
- **Other ways:** Inhalation of infected dust also transmitted TB.
- **Incubation period:** This may be weeks or months.

Clinical Features

- Chronic cough
- Continuous low grade fever
- Chest pain
- Hemoptysis
- Loss of weight

Control of TB

- **Sputum examination:** Sputum examination by direct microscopy is now considered by direct microscopy sputum should be examined from any patient presenting one or more of the following symptoms of respiratory disease.
  - Cough lasting more than 2 weeks
  - Continuous fever
  - Chest pain
  - Hemoptysis or spitting of blood.
- **Chemotherapy:** Chemotherapy has completely revolutionized the treatment of pulmonary tuberculosis. Every patient diagnosed by sputum examination should be put on multi drug treatment. If treatment is

irregular or interrupted, the patient may develop drug resistance and it becomes more difficult to treat the patient.

- **DOTS:** Direct observed treatment, short course. During intensive phase of chemotherapy, all the drugs are administered under direct supervision. DOTS will be given by peripheral health staff such as MPWs, teachers, Anganwadi workers, social workers, dais, ex-patients. They are known as DOTS agent.
- **BCG vaccination:** BCG should be given soon after birth. The dose of vaccine is 0.1 mL. For infants below the age of one month the dose is 0.05 mL.

  BCG does not give 100% protection against tuberculosis, the protection is about 80%. The immunity after BCG vaccination lasts for about 15 years.
- **Health education:** The health education program should be directed to motivating patients for undergoing regular treatment and follow-up, disposal of sputum and cooperations with agencies administering the program.

MEASLES

It is highly infectious disease caused by virus. It is characterized by fever, coughing, sneezing and running of nose, followed by a typical rash.

Mode of Transmissions

The mode of spread is from person-to-person. Directly through droplet infection, i.e. sneezing, talking, kissing. It also spreads by means of articles such as cups and spoons recently contaminated by the patient.

Incubation Period

10 to 14 days.

Clinical Features

- **Pre-eruptive stage:** The early symptoms are similar to those of severe cold namely fever, running nose, watery and red eyes, sneezing, small bluish-white spots on a red base known as koplik spots occur on the inner surface of the cheek during the prodromal period. These symptoms last for 3 to 4 days.
- **Eruptive stage:** About the 4th day of illness a typical dusky red macular rash appear, first on the face and neck, behind the ears and then spread down the body taking 2 to 3 days to progress to lower limbs.

The eruption lasts for about 5 to 6 days and gradually fades leaving dark pigmentation of the skin.

- **Prevention:**
  - **Measles vaccine:** A live measles vaccine is available. The child should be immunized according to immunization schedule at the age of 9 to 12 months.
- **Immunoglobulin:** Administration of human measles immunoglobulin in doses ranging from 250 to 750 mg can modify or prevent measles, if given within 3 days of contact.
- **Control:**
  - Isolation of the child as soon as sign of measles are evident.
  - Protection of the child's eyes from light or glare.
  - Disinfection of nose and throat discharges.
  - Immunization of susceptible children.

DENGUE FEVER

Dengue fever caused by arboviruses which capable of infecting humans and causing disease.

Types

1. Classical dengue fever
2. Dengue hemorrhagic fever without shock
3. Dengue hemorrhagic fever with shock.

- **Classical dengue fever:** It is also known as break-bone fever. It is an acute viral infection caused by at least 4 serotypes of dengue virus. The reservoir of infection is both man and mosquito. *Aedes aegypti* is the main vector.
- **Dengue hemorrhagic fever:** It is severe form of dengue fever caused by infection with more than one dengue virus.

Treatment

- The management of dengue fever is symptomatic and supportive.
- Bed rest is advisable during the acute febrile phase.
- Antipyretics or sponging are required to keep the body temperature below 40 °C.
- Aspirin should be avoided, particularly in areas where DHF is endemic.

QUALITIES OF COMMUNITY HEALTH NURSE

Refer Paper 2007 question no 4 (a).

Community Health Nursing
January 2013

Time: 3 Hours | **Maximum Marks: 75**

Note: *All questions are compulsory. Attempt all parts of questions in continuity.*

1. **Define the following terms:** **10×1=10**
   - (a) Pasteurization
   - (b) IUD
   - (c) Communicable disease
   - (d) Environment
   - (e) Health
   - (f) WHO
   - (g) Communication
   - (h) Immunity
   - (i) Pollution
   - (j) MMR

2. **(a) Define community health nursing.** **8+2=10**

   (b) Discuss the qualities of community health nursing.

3. **(a) Define primary health care.** **3×5=15**

   (b) Principles of primary health care

   (c) Discuss the functions of primary health center.

4. **Explain the following:** **3×5=15**
   - (a) Functions of protein
   - (b) Home visiting
   - (c) Principles of health education

5. **Write short notes on any five of the following:** **5×5=25**
   - (a) Anemia
   - (b) Bag technique
   - (c) Prevantion of water pollution
   - (d) Voluntary health agencies
   - (e) Advantages of breastfeeding
   - (f) Communication.

SOLVED QUESTION PAPER 2013

1. Define the following terms:

(a) Pasteurization	(b) IUD
(c) Communicable Disease	(d) Environment
(e) Health	(f) WHO
(g) Communication	(h) Immunity
(i) Pollution	(j) MMR.

PASTEURIZATION

The heating of milk to such temperature and for such period of time as are required to destroy any pathogens that may be present, while causing minimal change in the composition, flavors and nutritive value.

IUD

It is called intrauterine device. It is temporary method of family planning. It is used to control of conception by introducing a foreign body into the uterus such as copper - T.

COMMUNICABLE DISEASE

The disease which spreads from one person to another is called communicable disease for example tuberclosis.

ENVIRONMENT

The term environment implies all the extenal factors living and non-living, material and non-material, which surround human being.

HEALTH

According to WHO, it is defined as a state of complete physical, mental, social, spiritual well-being and not merely an absence of disease or infirmity.

WHO

World health organization is a specialized non-political, health agency of the united nations with headquarters at Geneva.

COMMUNICATION

It is defined as a process by which two or more persons exchange or share ideas, facts, feelings or expressions.

IMMUNITY

It is power of body to fight against infections.

POLLUTION

Pollution is a introduction of contaminants into the natural environment that cause adverse changes.

MMR

Maternal mortality rate is defined as death of a woman while pragnant or within 42 days of termination of pregnancy, from any cause related to pregnancy. It is measured by the formula:

$$\text{MMR} = \frac{\text{Total no. of female deaths due to complications of pregnancy, childbirth, or within 42 days of delivery from any puerperal causes in an area during a given year}}{\text{Total no. of live births in the same area and year}}$$

2. (a) Define community health nursing.

(b) Discuss the qualities of community health nursing.

COMMUNITY HEALTH NURSING

According to WHO, it refers to the health status of the members of the community, to the problems affecting their health and to the totality of health care provided to the community.

THE QUALITIES OF COMMUNITY HEALTH NURSING

Refer Paper November 2010, Q. No. 4(a).

3. (a) Define PHC

(b) Principles of PHC

(c) Discuss functions of PHC

PHC

Primary health centre provides essential health care made universally accessible to individuals and families in the community by means acceptable to them, through their full participation and at a cost that the community and country can afford.

PRINCIPLES OF PHC

Refer Paper November 2010, Q. No. 5(a).

FUNCTIONS OF PHC

Refer Paper September 2004, Q. No. 3(a).

4. Explain the following:
- (a) Functions of protein
- (b) Home visiting
- (c) Principles of health education

FUNCTIONS OF PROTEIN

Refer Paper November 2010, Q. No. 4(b).

HOME VISITING

It is a process through which a nurse or health personnel provides health care at door step. Means house to house care.

Principles → *Refer Paper 2006 Q. No. 4(c).*

PRINCIPLES OF HEALTH EDUCATION

Refer Important Theory, Q. No. 6.

5. Write short notes on any five of the following:
- (a) Anemia
- (b) Bag Technique
- (c) Prevention of water pollution
- (d) Voluntary health agencies
- (e) Advantages of breastfeeding
- (f) Communication

ANEMIA

It means lack of hemoglobin level in the body.

Causes

- Due to deficiency of iron
- Due to inadequate take of diet
- Due to deficiency of folic acid
- Deficiency of Vit. B12

Signs and Symptoms

- Weakness
- Inability to do work
- Diginess
- Fatigue
- Lethargy

Prevention of Anemia

Refer Paper 2009, Q. No. 6(c).

BAG TECHNIQUE

Community bag is a bag which is carried by a nurse during home visiting. Community bag contains all the articles, which are required for nursing procedures during home visiting.

Procedures of Bag Technique

- Spread the newspaper or plastic sheet on a flat surface in clean area and place the bag on it.
- It should keep away soap and water each time before opening the bag.
- Wash hand with soap and water each time before opening the bag.
- Remove only the needed articles.
- Carry out the nursing procedure.
- Wash and boil the instruments after finishing the work.
- Wash hand, open the bag and replace the articles them in the bag.
- If boiling is not possible, place them in a separate bag.
- Burn the soil dressing.
- Fold the used newspaper with used side inside and keep it in outer pocket.
- Record the procedure on notebook.

PREVENTION OF WATER POLLUTION

Various methods are used to prevent water pollution:

- **Selection of source of water:** Select the ground or other water which is away from human excreta.
- Allways cover the water ponds/tank and other drinkable water.
- Appropriate water treatment requirements and necessary pollution control measures to protect raw water resources.
- Sanitation measures are used to protect the water from getting polluted.
- **National water supply:** The national water supply and sanitation programme was launched in 1954 by the Government of India as part of the health plan to assist the states to provide adquate water supply and sanitation facilities in the entire country.

- **Health education:** All the preventive measures not successful without awareness of public. For this, only one method is useful that is health education.

VOLUNTARY HEALTH AGENCIES

There are various nongovernmental voluntary health agencies at the national and international level, which contribute towards health, welfare and developmental aspects as per requirements during emergencies and normal situation.

Voluntary Health Agencies Include:

- Indian Red Cross Society
- Hind Kusht Nivaran Sangh
- Indian Council for Child Welfare
- Tuberculosis Association of India
- Bharat Sevak Samaj
- Central Social Welfare Board
- The Kasturba Memorial Fund
- Family Planning Association of India
- All India Women's Conference
- All India Blind Relief Society

Functions

- **Supplementing** the work of Govt. agencies.
- It helps in research activities such as family planning.
- **Education:** There is unlimited scope for health education in India.
- **Demonstration:** By putting up demonstration and experimental projects, the voluntary effort on the part of people.
- Guiding the work of Government Agencies.
- **Advancing Health Legislation:** The voluntary agencies can also mobilize public opinion and advance legislation on health matters for the benefit of the whole community.

ADVANTAGES OF BREASTFEEDING

Refer Paper 2009, Q. No. 6(a).

COMMUNICATION

Communication can be regarded as a process by which two or more persons exchange ideas, facts, feelings or expressions.

Process and its Importance → *Refer Paper 2009, Q. No. 5(a).*

Community Health Nursing
January 2012

Time: 3 Hours **Maximum Marks: 75**

Note: *Attempt all the questions. Attempt all parts of questions at same places.*

1. **Define the following terms:** **5×2=10**
   (a) Levels of prevention
   (b) Malnutrition
   (c) Communication
   (d) Community health
   (e) Immunity
2. **(a) What is home visiting?** **3+7=10**
   (b) Explain principles of home visiting.
3. **(a) Define epidemiology.** **3+5+7=15**
   (b) Write aims of epidemiology.
   (c) Describe the tools of measurement in epidemiology?
4. **Describe in detail any three:** **3×5=15**
   (a) Standing orders
   (b) Types and uses of record
   (c) Immunization schedule
   (d) Qualities and functions of community health nurse.
5. **Write short notes on any five.** **5×5=25**
   (a) Factors affecting selection and planning of meal
   (b) Principles of cooking food
   (c) Barriers of communication
   (d) Water-borne diseases
   (e) Importance of environmental health
   (f) Methods of health education.

SOLVED QUESTION PAPER 2012

1. Define the following terms:

(a) Levels of prevention
(b) Malnutrition
(c) Communication
(d) Community health
(e) Immunity

LEVELS OF PREVENTION

In modern way, the concept of prevention becomes broad based. It has become customary to define prevention in terms of three levels:

1. Primary prevention
2. Secondary prevention
3. Tertiary prevention

MALNUTRITION

It is a condition, which occurs when the body does not get the proper kind of food in the amounts needed for maintaining health.

COMMUNICATION

It is a defined as a process by which two or more persons exchange or share ideas, facts, feelings or expressions.

COMMUNITY HEALTH

Community health refers to the health status of the members of the community, to the problems affecting their health, and to the totality of health care provided to the community.

IMMUNITY

It is the power of body to fight against infection.

2. (a) What is home visiting?
(b) Explain the principles of home visiting.

HOME VISITING

It means visiting the family at their place to assess the health needs, to provide services such as preventive, promotive, curative or rehabilitative services at their door-step by community health nurse or health worker.

PRINCIPLES OF HOME VISITING

Refer Paper 2006, Q. No. 4(c).

3. (a) Define epidemiology.
(b) Write aims of epidemiology.
(c) Describe the tools of measurement in epidemiology.

DEFINE EPIDEMIOLOGY

According to US National Institute of Health

Epidemiology is the study of the patterns, causes and control of disease in groups of people.

Or

Epidemiology is concerned with the pattern of disease occurrence in human population and of the factors that influence these patterns.

AIMS OF EPIDEMIOLOGY

- To determine the frequency and distribution of a disease in a population.
- To identify the etiology to achieve control over the disease.
- To assess the economic effects of a disease and to analyze the costs and economic benefits of alternative control programs.
- To describe the distribution and magnitude of health and disease problems in human population.
- To identify etiological factors in the pathogenesis of diseases.
- To provide the data essential to planning, implementation and evaluation of services for prevention, control and treatment of diseases and to setting up of priorities among these services.

BASIC TOOLS OF MEASUREMENT IN EPIDEMIOLOGY

Epidemiology focuses on basic tools of measurement by which mortality and morbidity in population is measured, i.e. rates, ratio of populations.

Following are measured in epidemiology:

- Mortality
- Morbidity
- Disability
- Nationality
- Attributes of disease: Present or absent
- Medical needs

- Health care facilities
- Utilization of health services
- Environmental factors suspected of causing disease
- Demographic variables
- Psychosocial aspects of health.

The magnitude of above all is expressed by epidemiologist in the form of:

- Rate
- Ratio
- Proportion.

Example of Rates

- Mortality rate
- Morbidity rate
- Crude birth rate
- Specific rate.

Example of Ratio

- Sex ratio
- Doctor, population ratio
- Child, women ratio.

Example of Proportion

- Proportion of scabies
- Proportion of utilization of health services.

Rate

A rate measures the occurrence of some particular events in a population during a given time period. Rate indicates the change in some events that take place in a population over a period of time.

For Example

- Death rate
- Birth rate
- Specific rate.

Elements of Rate

- Numerator
- Denominator

- Time specification
- Multiplier.

$$\text{Crude death rate} = \frac{\text{No. of healths in one year}}{\text{Mid-year population}} \times 100$$

In above rate, numerator is the number of deaths.

- Denominator is midyear population
- One year is time specification
- Multiplier is 1,000.

Ratio

Ratio can express a relation in size between two random quantities. In other words, ratio is the result of dividing one quantity by another.

$$A : B \text{ or } \frac{A}{B}$$

Proportion

It is also a ratio that indicates the relation in magnitude of a part of the whole proportion. It is expressed as a percentage, e.g.

$$\frac{\text{The number of children with scabies at a certain time}}{\text{The total number of children in village at the same time}} \times 100$$

4. Describe in detail any three:

(a) Standing orders
(b) Types and uses of record
(c) Immunization schedule
(d) Qualities and functions of community health nurse

STANDING ORDERS

Standing orders are specific instructions issued to CHN by authorized committee or agency regarding treatment for certain conditions, which the nurse may meet in home or in the community.

Purposes

- To handle emergencies, especially in rural areas, in the absence of doctors
- To reduce danger in acute conditions
- To promote health services in the community.

Policy of the Agencies

Each hospital or agency can formulate its own standing orders for CHN according to the conditions in the community. The standing orders are reviewed periodically by medical nursing personnel, jointly updated or modified.

Nursing Responsibilities

- Proper recording
- Ascertain complaints, onset and duration
- Large medical care and reassure the family carry-out standing instructions according to the manual
- Notify appropriate authority for common diseases
- Referral services to be carried out
- Follow-up.

Limitations

The CHN should remember carefully that she is not a doctor in carrying out these orders on regular basis.
- Services should be limited.
- She can provide Rx only in emergencies or in absence of doctor.
- She should consult the medical officer at the time of doubt and difficulty.

Every health service should issue standing orders to meet the needs of the services in the field.

TYPES AND USES OF RECORD

Refer Paper 2007 Q. No. 4 (c) and Important Theory Q. No. 10.

IMMUNIZATION SCHEDULE

Refer Important Theory Q. No. 12.

QUALITIES AND FUNCTIONS OF COMMUNITY HEALTH NURSE

Refer Paper 2010 Q. No. 4(a) and Paper 2006, Q. No. 5(d).

5. Write short notes on any five.

(a) Factors affecting selection and planning of meal
(b) Principles of cooking food
(c) Barriers of communication
(d) Waterborne diseases

(e) Importance of environmental health
(f) Methods of health education.

FACTORS AFFECTING SELECTION AND PLANNING OF MEAL

There are various social, religious and economic factors influencing nutritional needs of people. Various factors are:

- Racial habits
- Religious practices
- Requirements of the family group
- Economic factors.

Racial Habits

There are various groups, communities and races in a country like India and they choose as per their racial habits and the availability of food. Also the climate and soil of a particular area affects the nutritional habits.

Religious Practices

India is a religious country and people practice different religious laws, e.g. muslims and jews do not eat pork whereas Hindus do not consume beef. Adequate planning must be done as many are vagetarian and other nonvegetarian. Those who do not eat eggs and meat must plan their menu as per the exchange list.

Requirement of Family

It includes composition of family, occupation and special requirements of vulnerable groups such as children, pregnant ladies and lactating mothers. If the family is large, special consideration must be given for each age group for their nutritional needs. Menu planning is done as per recommended dietary allowances.

Economic Factors

This factor is most important one, as today, each and every food commodity is to be purchased and if there is less money, there will be lack of various nutrients in diet. This means that more foods, which are energy-yielding are consumed over the foods which provides growth and species of body which as a result, lead to malnutrition. The balanced diet is more costly for a common person to afford. Ignorance and pooverty are the main factors leading to malnutrition, and therefore, it can be concluded that the nutritional efficiency of a country depends upon the economic factors of a country.

PRINCIPLES OF COOKING FOOD

Refer Paper 2007, Q. No. 3(d).

BARRIERS OF COMMUNICATION

Refer Paper 2007, Q. No. 5(b).

WATERBORNE DISEASES

Refe Paper 2008, Q. No. 2.

IMPORTANCE OF ENVIRONMENTAL HEALTH

Much of ill-health in India is due to poor environmental sanitation, that is, unsafe water, polluted soil, unhygienic disposal of human excreta and refuse, poor housing, insects and rodents. Air pollution is also a growing concern in many cities. The high death rate, infant mortality rate, sickness rate and poor standard of health are, in fact, largely due to defective environmental sanitation.

Improvement of environmental sanitation is, therefore, crucial for the prevention of diseases and promotion of health of individuals and communities. Since more than 70% of the population of India live in rural areas, the problem is one of rural sanitation. The first step in only health program is the elimination through environmental control of those factors which are harmful to health.

METHODS OF HEALTH EDUCATION

There are various methods of health education. These have been classified as below:

One-way or Didactic Methods

- Lecture
- Films
- Charts
- Flannelgraph
- Exhibits
- Flash cards.

Two-way or Socratic Methods

- Group discussion
- Panel discussion

- Symposium
- Workshop
- Role playing
- Demonstration.

Health education is mainly carried out at 3 main levels:

1. Individuals
2. Group
3. General public

All above methods used for Group Teaching:

Individual Health Education

Doctors or nurses who are in direct contact with patients and their relatives have opportunities for much individual health education. The topic selected should be relevant to the situation. For instance, a mother who has come for delivery should be told about child birth—not about malaria eradication.

In this method, we can reach only small group or individual member.

Method for General Public Education

We employ 'Mass Media Communication'.

For Example

- Posters
- Health magazines
- Press
- Films
- Radio
- Museums
- TV
- Indigenous medico

They are very useful in reaching large member of people with whom otherwise there could be no contact.

Community Health Nursing
November 2010

Time: 3 Hours | **Maximum Marks: 75**

Note: *Attempt all the questions and their parts in continuity.*

1. Define the following terms: 5×1=5

(a) Balanced diet
(b) Communication
(c) PEM
(d) Pasteurization
(e) Metabolism

2. Fill in the blanks: 5×1=5

(a) Night blindness is caused by the deficiency of vitamin________.
(b) ____________ is classified as body building food.
(c) Deafness is caused by ____________ pollution.
(d) 1 gm of fat yields ____________ calories.
(e) Typhoid is a ________________ borne disease.

3. Write down the following: 4×5=20

(a) Purpose of home visiting
(b) Principles of cooking
(c) Functions of primary health center
(d) Household methods of storing food

4. Explain the following: 3×5=15

(a) Qualities of community health nursing
(b) Functions of protein
(c) Sources of vitamins

5. Describe the following: 3×5=15

(a) Principles of primary health care
(b) Role of female health worker at subcenter level
(c) Food adulteration

6. Write short notes on any three of the following: 5×3=15

(a) Immunization schedule
(b) Disease cycle

(c) Indicators of health
(d) Importance of records
(e) Community health nursing process

SOLVED QUESTION PAPER 2010

1. Define the following terms:
(a) Balanced diet
(b) Communication
(c) PEM
(d) Pasteurization
(e) Metabolism

BALANCED DIET

Balanced diet is the one which consists of all the required nutrients in correct or adequate amount for proper maintenance and regulation of body functions.

COMMUNICATION

Communication is defined as a process by which two or more persons exchange or share ideas, facts, feeling or expressions.

PEM

It is the common nutritional problem among the preschoolers. It affects on growth and development of a child. It causes two diseases—kwashiorkor and marasmus.

PASTEURIZATION

The heating of milk to such temperatures and for such periods of time as are required to destroy any pathogens that may be present while causing minimal changes in the composition, flavor and nutritive value.

METABOLISM

It is defined as all biochemical reactions occurring in the body.

2. Fill in the blanks:
(a) Night blindness is caused by the deficiency of vitamin ________________.
(b) ________________ is classified as body building food.

(c) Deafness is caused by ____________ pollution.
(d) 1 gm of fat yields ____________ calories.
(e) Typhoid is a ____________________ borne disease.

FILL IN THE BLANKS

(a) Night blindness is caused by the deficiency of vitamin **...A...** .
(b) **....Protein....** is classified as body building food.
(c) Deafness is caused by........**Noise**..... pollution.
(d) 1 gm of fat yields ......**9**....... calories.
(e) Typhoid is a .....**water**....borne disease.

3. Write down the following:

(a) Purpose of home visiting.
(b) Principles of cooking.
(c) Functions of primary health center.
(d) Household methods of storing food.

PURPOSES OF HOME VISITING

- It is a routine part of a planned visiting program by community health personnel.
- It helps to investigate the sources of infectious diseases.
- To do follow-up on some problems identified, in industry or hospital, school and health centers.
- To assess the nutritional immunization status and environmental hazards.
- To give health education to the individual, family and community.
- To supervise and guide other health workers.

PRINCIPLES OF COOKING

Some of the basic principles of cooking must be kept in mind to prevent under-nutrition and over-nutrition. Some of which are enlisted below.

- Food must not be overcooked or undercooked to prevent the loss of essential nutrients and latter to control microbes count.
- In must be as per climatic conditions and seasoning must be done with suitable condiments.
- There should be variety in cooking. Same pattern of cooking may lead to rejection of some nutritious foods.
- Excessive use of condiments like salt and red pepper may lead to common problems like hypertension and piles.

- It must be done in a hygienic place. Handling and storing of food must also be done in some hygienic place.

FUNCTIONS OF PRIMARY HEALTH CENTER

- Medical care
- MCH, family planning and welfare
- School health services
- Improvement in environmental sanitation
- Control and surveillance of communicable disease
- Control/eradication of national health programs
- Collection and reporting of vital statistics
- Health education
- Training of auxiliary health personnel
- Nutritional services
- Immunization services
- Referral services.

HOUSEHOLD METHODS OF STORING FOOD

Cold Storage

The home refrigerator has now made it possible to store and preserve a variety of foods. Fruits and vegetables should be kept just above freezing point. Meat is kept at much lower temperature. It prevents the growth of microorganisms.

Drying and Dehydration

Drying removes water and in the absence of water microorganism cannot grow. Fruits, fish and meat are preserved by drying.

Smoking

Smoke which contains phenols helps in food preservation.

Salting and Pickling

Salt is preservative, by adding certain condiments and spices along with salt certain foods like mangoes, vegetables, meat and fish may be preserved.

Canning

Home canning is generally not recommended unless the technique employed is foolproof.

4. Explain the following:

(a) Qualities of community health nurse

(b) Functions of protein.

(c) Sources of vitamins.

QUALITIES OF COMMUNITY HEALTH NURSE

- A qualified community health nurse is one who has undergone basic general nursing, midwifery training and post-basic education in community health nursing.
- A community health nurse must have interest in people and in understanding human behavior.
- Sincerity and empathy are basic qualities of a nurse.
- She is honest, charitable, resourceful, cooperative and takes responsibilities with initiative, are also qualities of a nurse.
- Minimum essential skills of a nurse are observation, communication, interviewing and supportive and technical skills.

FUNCTIONS OF PROTEIN

- Proteins help in synthesis of enzymes, immunoglobulins, plasma proteins and hormones.
- Proteins help in growth and repair of body tissues.
- Proteins are secondary sources of energy during deficiency of carbohydrates and fats. It provide 4 kilo calories of energy.
- Proteins supply the material for building and continuous replacement of cell proteins.
- Proteins are the chief sole matter of muscle organs of endocrine glands.
- They are also component of skin, nails hair, blood cells and serum and the matrix of bone and teeth.
- Except bile and urine, every living cell and body fluids contain proteins.
- They are important for body regulatory mechanisms like formation of hemoglobin and antibodies.

SOURCES OF VITAMINS

- **Sources of vitamin 'A':** Milk, butter, cheese, egg yolk, fish, liver oils, green and yellow vegetables.

- **Sources of vitamin 'D':** Fish, liver oils, milk, cheese, egg yolk, irradiated 7 dehydrocholesterol in human skin.
- **Sources of vitamin 'E':** Egg yolk, milk, butter, green vegetables, nuts.
- **Sources of vitamin 'K':** Leafy vegetables, fish, liver, fruits.
- **Sources of vitamin B_1:** Yeast, liver germ of cereals, nuts pulses, rice, polishing, egg yolk, liver, legumes.
- **Sources of vitamin B_2:** Liver, yeast, milk, eggs, green vegetables, fish.
- **Sources of B_6:** Meat, liver, vegetables, bran of cereals, egg yolk, brans.
- **Sources of B_{12}:** Liver, milk, moulds.
- **Sources of folic acid:** Dark green vegetables, liver, kidney, eggs, synthesized in colon.
- **Sources of niacin:** Yeast, fish, pulses, whole meal cereals.
- **Sources of pantothenic acid:** Yeast, egg yolk, fresh vegetables.
- **Sources of biotin:** Yeast, liver, kidney, pulses, nuts.
- **Sources of vitamin 'C':** Citrus fruits, green vegetables, potatoes, liver and glandular tissue in animals.

5. **Describe the following:**
   (a) Principles of primary health care.
   (b) Role of female health worker at subcenter level.
   (c) Food adulteration.

PRINCIPLES OF PRIMARY HEALTH CARE

- **Equitable distribution:** Primary health care services must be shared equally by all people irrespective of their ability to pay.
- **Community participation:** Primary health care is for the people, by the people. The local community must participate in the planning, implementation and maintenance of health services.
- **Coverage and accessibility:** Primary health care implies providing health care services to all, which are required by them. The care has to be appropriate and adequate in amount to satisfy the essential health needs of the people and has to be provided by methods acceptable to them.
- **Intersectoral coordination:** Primary health care requires joint efforts of other health-related sectors such as agriculture, animal husbandry, food industry, housing, social welfare, public work and communication, etc.
- **Appropriate health technology:** Technology that is scientific, adaptable to local need and socially acceptable instead of costly methods, equipment and technology.

- **Referral system:** Referral system would be desirable to develop referring from one level to another with laid down procedures and policies.
- **Logistics of supply:** The logistics of supply include planning and budgeting for the supplies, required procurement or manufacture, storage distribution and control.
- **The physical facilities:** The physical facilities for primary health care need to be simple and clean. It should have a waiting area with toilet facility.

ROLE OF FEMALE HEALTH WORKER AT SUBCENTER LEVEL

- She provides reproductive and child health care services at subcenter level.
- She participates in family planning programs, which are provided at subcenter level.
- She provides health education to the people about MTP Act and its benefits, etc.
- She is notifying the communicable disease in the area and provides preventive and curative services to control these diseases.
- She has participation in training programs for dais and other assistant health workers.
- She is maintaines health records of people and the health services which are provided to the public.
- She also submits its report about health services to the authority.
- She provides primary health care to the community.
- She acts as a coordinator between team members.
- She acts as an educator. She provides health education and information to the people.

FOOD ADULTERATION

Food adulteration is a malpractice in which the food quality is substandarized by many subpractices such as:

- Mixing up of food products with contaminants
- Substitution of quality nutrients with substandard adulterants
- Abstraction of nutrients
- Concealing the quality
- Putting up decomposed foods for sale
- Misbranding
- Giving false labels
- Addition of toxicants.

Adulteration, various in different places and in different food commodities, some of the examples are illustrated below:

Milk

Removal of fat, addition of water, addition of starch to increase its consistency.

Ghee

Pure ghee is adulterated with dalda and animal's fat such as pig's fat.

Rice and Wheat

These are adulterated with mud, stones to increase their bulk.

Flour

Wheat flour is mixed with cheaper flour and soap stone power.

Pulses

Chemical substances are added to improve the appearance of old stock; stone chips are added to increase bulk.

Honey

It is adulterated with sugar and boiled with empty beehives.

Tea and Coffee

Tea leaves are adulterated with old tea leaves, leather and saw dust coffee is adulterated with chicory.

Medicines

Drugs are adulterated with substandard chemicals, which reduce their potentialities and efficiency.

6. Write short notes on any three of the following.

(a) Immunization schedule
(b) Disease cycle
(c) Indicators of health
(d) Importance of records
(e) Community health nursing process.

IMMUNIZATION SCHEDULE

Refer Important Theory, Q. No. 12.

DISEASE CYCLE

The course of most communicable disease is marked by certain stages. These stages are:

- **Incubation period:** This is time interval between the entry of the disease agent in the body and manifestation of clinical signs and symptoms.
- **Prodromal period**: This is a short period ranging from 1 to 4 days and is marked by vague signs and symptoms i.e. clinical diagnosis is usually not possible.
- **Fastigium:** This represents the height of the disease, signs and symptoms are clear. The patient is confined to bed. Clinical diagnosis is possible.
- **Defervescence:** The patient begins to feel better. The body defense (immunity) begins to respond.
- **Convalescence:** The patient's recovery is established, he is improving fast.
- **Deinfection:** The patient recovers from illness.

INDICATORS OF HEALTH

Definition

Health indicators are the measures of the health status of community by which health of that community is known.

Indicators of health are:

- **Mortality indicators:** It means the rate at which people are dying.
- **Crude death rate:** Defined as the number of deaths per 1,000 population per year in a given community.

$$\text{Crude death rate} = \frac{\text{No. of deaths during a given year}}{\text{Mid year population of same year}} \times 100$$

- **Infant mortality rate:** The number if deaths under 1 year of age per 1,000 in a given year to the total number of live births in the same year.
- **Child mortality indicators:** It is defined as the number of deaths at age 1 to 4 years in a given year per 1,000 children in that age group at mid-point of the same year. Infant mortality is excluded.

Child mortality rate =

$$\frac{\text{No. of deaths at - 4 year of age in given year}}{\text{Total children 1 - 4 year at midpoint of same year}} \times 100$$

- **Under 5 mortality:** It is defined as the proportion of total deaths occurring in the under five age group.
  Under five mortality =

$$\frac{\text{Total no. of deaths in under five years of age}}{\text{Total no. of children under five years of age}} \times 100$$

- **Maternal mortality rate:** It is defined as the number of deaths among women of reproductive age in a year per 1,000, live births in the same area and year.

$$\text{MMR} = \frac{\text{No. of new and old cases of specific disease during a given time period}}{\text{Popuation at risk during that period}} \times 1{,}000$$

- **Disease specific mortality rate:** It is defined as the number of deaths due to specific disease in a given year per 1,000 mid-year population in the same year.
- **Expectation of life:** It is defined as the average number of years that will be lived by those born alive into a population if the current age specific mortality rate persists.

Morbidity Indicators

The morbidity indicators are used for assessing ill-health in a community, e.g.:

a. **Incidence rate:** It is defined as the number of new cases occurring in a defined population during a specified period of time.

$$\text{Incidence rate} = \frac{\text{No. of new and old cases of specific disease during a given time period}}{\text{Popuation at risk during that period}} \times 1{,}000$$

b. **Prevalence rate:** It is defined as a number of old and new cases occurring in a defined population during a specified period of time.

$$\text{Prevalence} = \frac{\text{No. of new and old cases of specific disease during a given time period}}{\text{Popuation at risk during that period}} \times 1{,}000$$

- **Disability indicators:** Disability rates related to illness are used as supplement morbidity and mortality rate (common), e.g. are
  - Even type indicator
  - Person type indicator.
- **Nutritional status indicators:** There are three main nutritional indicators such as anthropometric, height and prevalence of nutrition. It is used to measure health status of the children.
- **Health care delivery indicators:**
  - Doctor population ratio
  - Doctor nurse ratio
  - Population bed ratio.
- **Socioeconomic indicators:**
  - Rate of population increase
  - Level of employment
  - Dependency ratio
  - Family size
  - Per capita 'calorie' availability
  - Literacy rate.
- **Other indicators:**
  - Sociol indicators
  - Basic need indictors
  - Health for all indicators

IMPORTANCE OF RECORDS

- Effective means of communication
- Help in providing best possible services to the individual, family and community
- Can save effort and money
- Useful in research
- Can be useful as an instrument of health education
- Provides a basis for long-and-short-term learning.
- Helps to organize the work.

COMMUNITY HEALTH NURSING PROCESS

Refer Paper October 2007, Q. No. 6(a).

Community Health Nursing
November 2009

Time: 3 Hours **Maximum Marks: 75**

Note: *Attempt all questions and their parts in continuity.*

1. **Define the following terms:** 5×1=5
   (a) Epidemic
   (b) Environment
   (c) Community health
   (d) Records
   (e) Disinfection
2. **Fill in the blanks:** 5×1=5
   (a) Stagnant water is a breeding place for ________.
   (b) Goiter is caused by deficiency of ________.
   (c) Fat is classified as________ food.
   (d) __________ is a poor source of iron.
   (e) One gram of carbohydrate yields _________ calories. 3×5=15
3. **Describe the following:**
   (a) Modes of transmission of communicable diseases.
   (b) Principles of primary health care.
   (c) Role of community health nurse in the PHC.
4. **Write down the following:** 4×5=20
   (a) Methods of food preservation
   (b) Functions of protein
   (c) Advantages of records and reports
   (d) Purification of water
   (e) Prevention of air pollution.
5. **Explain the following:** 3×5 =15
   (a) Process of communication and its importance.
   (b) Methods of disinfection.
   (c) Functions of family planning clinic.
6. **Write short notes on any three:** 3×5=15
   (a) Breastfeeding (b) Health team
   (c) Prevention of anemia (d) Disease cycle.

SOLVED QUESTION PAPER 2009

1. Define the following terms:
(a) Epidemic
(b) Environment
(c) Community health
(d) Records
(e) Disinfection

EPIDEMIC (EPI–UPON, DEMOS–PEOPLE)

An outbreak of disease in a community in excess of 'Normal expectation' and derived from a common source.

ENVIRONMENT

The term 'Environment' includes all the external factors, living and non-living materials and nonmaterial—which surround man.

COMMUNITY HEALTH

Community health refers to the health status of the members of the community, to the problems affecting their health, and to the totality of health care provided to the community.

RECORDS

Records are written and legal documents in which there is collection of information about patient.

DISINFECTION

Killing of infectious agents outside the human body by direct exposure to chemical or physical agent.

2. Fill in the blanks:
(a) Stagnant water is a breeding place for ________.
(b) Goiter is caused by deficiency of ________.
(c) Fat is classified as________ food.
(d) ________ is a poor source of iron.
(e) One gram of carbohydrate yields ________ calories.

FILL IN THE BLANKS

(a) Stagnant water is a breeding place for M**osquito.**
(b) Goiter is caused by deficiency of **Iodine.**
(c) Fat is classified as **Energy-yielding** food.
(d) **Milk** is a poor source of iron.
(e) One gram of carbohydrate yields **4 k** calories.

3. Describe the following:
(a) Modes of transmission of communicable disease.
(b) Principles of primary health care.
(c) Role of community health nurse in the PHC.

MODES OF COMMUNICABLE DISEASE TRANSMISSION

Modes of Transmission

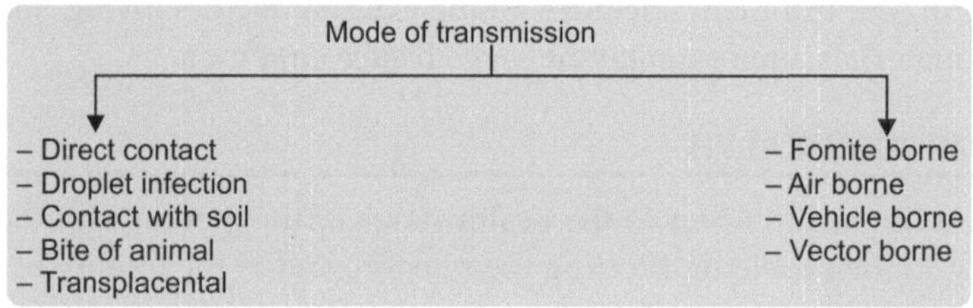

DIRECT TRANSMISSION

Direct Contact

Some diseases are transmitted directly from person to person by direct contact, touching and by kissing, etc. Diseases spread by direct contact are AIDS, scabies, etc.

Droplet Infection

Fine drops of secretion from infected person spread disease, e.g. by sneezing, coughing, spitting, singing and talking, etc. and diseases spread through droplet transmission are common cold, diphtheria, tuberculosis, etc.

Contact with Soil

Some disease agents are acquired by dirty soil. For example, tetanus, hookworm, etc.

Inoculated Directly in Skin or Mucosa

When the infectious agent inoculated directly into skin, e.g. dog bite. Rabies is caused due to bite of rabid animal.

Transplacental Transmission

Some diseases spread through placenta from mother to fetus, e.g. AIDS. It is also called vertical transmission of disease.

INDIRECT TRANSMISSION

Airborne

The infectious agent which comes out from infected person by different ways, if inhaled by healthy person, it causes infection.

Vehicle Borne

The chief vehicles are food, water, milk, blood, serum, etc. The diseases transmitted by food, water, milk are food poisoning, cholera, etc. and disease spreads by blood contact is hepatitis.

Vector Borne

Malaria, filaria, kala-azar are diseases spread by insects. They are called vector-borne diseases.

Fomites Borne

Fomites are articles other than food and drinking. The articles which are infected by patient and used by healthy persons cause disease. Article, e.g. pencil, books, clothes, etc.

PRINCIPLES OF PRIMARY HEALTH CARE

Equitable Distribution

Primary health care must be shared equally by all people irrespective of their ability to pay, i.e. rich or poor urban or rural people.

Community Participation

Primary health care is for the people, by the people. The local community must participate in the planning, implementation, and maintenance of health services.

Appropriate Technology

Use those methods which are socially acceptable and affordable by all.

Prevention

The emphasis is on prevention. It runs through all the elements of primary health care.

Multisectoral Approach

Primary health care is that which cannot be achieved by the health sector alone. It requires joint efforts of other health-related sectors such as agriculture, education and social welfare, etc.

ROLE OF COMMUNITY HEALTH NURSE IN THE PHC

- Community health nurses work with population, community, family and individual.
- Assessing the health status of individuals and communities.
- Mobilizing community involvement.
- Providing integrated health care including the treatment of emergencies and making referrals.
- Maintaining epidemiological surveillance.
- Training and supervising health workers.
- Collaborating with other development sectors.
- Monitoring progress in primary health care.
- She focuses on assessment of the impact of the socioeconomical and cultural factors affecting health.
- She works in school where primary goal is health education and disease prevention.

4. Write down the following:

(a) Methods of food preservation.
(b) Functions of proteins.
(c) Advantages of records and reports.
(d) Purification of water.
(e) Prevention of air pollution

METHODS OF FOOD PRESERVATION

Household Methods

- **Cold storage:** The home refrigerator has now made it possible to store and preserve a variety of foods. There is no growth of food poisoning organisms at this low temperature.

- **Drying or dehydration:** Drying removes water, and in the absence of water, microorganism cannot grow. Fruits, fish, meat are preserved by this method.
- **Smoking:** Phenols used in smoking for preservation of food.
- **Salting and pickling:** By adding some condiments with salt preserve food; mangoes, meat, fish, vegetables are preserved by this method.
- **Canning:** It is less used method in house storage.

Commercial Methods

- **Canning:** Before canning, sterilize food at high temperature (135°–175°C) for short time and then cooled and filled in pre-sterilized containers.
- **Freezing:** A number of foods are preserved by this method and stored for long time.
- **Chemicals:** Some chemicals like benzoic acid and sodium benzoate are used; but their uses are strictly limited by government.
- **Irradiation:** Microorganisms are destroyed by gamma rays. Wheat, potatoes, and onion may be preserved by irradiation.

FUNCTIONS OF PROTEINS

- **Growth and development:** Proteins provide body-building material. So proteins are essential for growth and development.
- **For repair of body tissues and their maintenance:** Proteins repair the body tissues, which break down due to any injury and help in maintaining body tissues in good condition.
- **For synthesis of antibodies, enzymes and hormones:** Antibodies, enzymes and hormones contain protein and all these are essential to protect body from infection.

ADVANTAGES OF RECORDS AND REPORTS

Records are written documents in which is collected information about an individual and family. This information includes socioeconomical, psychological and environmental factors of patient and family.
Records are maintained by nurses, doctors and by other health workers, about clients.

- It helps in providing best possible service to the individual, family and community.
- It provides basis for short and long-term planning.
- It prevents duplication of services and helps to follow-up service effectively.

- It helps the nurse to evaluate the care and teaching, which she has given.
- Records helps to become aware of and recognise the health needs of the individual and family.
- Records can be used as a teaching tool to the individual and family.
- Records help in diagnosis, treatment and evaluation for the doctors.
- Records help to identify families needing services, and those prepared to accept help.
- It helps the nurse to judge the quality of work done.
- It can save effort and money.
- It is useful in research.
- The health workers can organize their work or make the most effective use of the time.
- Reports are the effective method of communication between the members of the health team. Reports should be truthful, accurate, clear, brief and complete.
- Good reports will indicate the efficiency of health team in carrying out their work.

PURIFICATION OF WATER

- Water available in nature from surface or underground source is described as 'raw' water. It requires purification before it can be supplied to the community.
- In natural purification, physical, chemical and biological processes take place. First store the water from various sources.
  - **Physical process:** Physical action of stored water helps to settle down the impurities in 24 hours due to gravity. This water becomes clear. This allows sunlight to penetrate and reduce the work of filter.
  - **Chemical process:** Aerobic bacteria oxidize the organic matter present in stored water utilizing dissolved oxygen.
  - **Biological process:** Biological process during storage helps in reducing the amount of bacteria present in water. Pathogens die in 5 to 7 days of storage.

Filtration

Filtration is second stage of water purification. Ninty eight to ninety nine percent of bacteria first are removed by filtration. There are two types of filters which are commonly used:

- Slow sand or biological filter
- Rapid sand or mechanical filter.

Slow Sand Filter

It was first used in 1804 in Scotland and accepted as a standard method of water purification.

Advantages

- Equipment needed is simple
- Supervision is simple
- Quality of filtered water is high
- Simple to operate.

Elements

- **Storage:** First store the water in settlement tanks for 1 to 2 days where natural purification takes place.
- **Sand bed:** In next step the stored water is admitted into slow sand filter where sand is main filtering medium. In this first place, bricks or stone layer at the bottom 6 to 12 inches thick, above this another layer of gravel 12 inches deep. Above this 3 to 5 feet fine sand is placed. Above the sand, 4 to 5 feet water is allowed to stand for filtering the bottom of the bed are attached pipes which collect the filtered water.

Under Drainage System

It consist of pipes which serve the outlet for filtered water. It consists of three elements—supernatant water, sand bed and under drainage system.

Filter Control

The purpose of these devices is to maintain a constant rate of filtration, filter may run for weeks even months without cleaning.

Disadvantages

- A filtration is open, possibility of contamination is more.
- Large area is required.
- Less feasibility in operation.

Rapid Sand Filtration

Rapid sand filtration was first used in 1885 in USA. It's of two types:

- Gravity type
- Pressure type

Steps of Rapid Sand Filtration

- Coagulation
- Mixing
- Flocculation
- Sedimentation
- Filtration.

Coagulation

The raw water is first treated with a chemical coagulant such as alum for removal of turbidity and color. The amount of alum to be added can be between 5 and 40 mg per liter depending upon the turbidity.

Mixing

After addition of alum the water is mixed in mixing chamber.

Flocculation

Then the water is passed into the flocculation chamber for 30 minutes.

Sedimentation

Coagulated water is led into sedimentation tank for a period of 2 to 6 hours, the water now looks much clear in appearance.

Filtration

In this process, water is purified up to 99%.

Disinfection

Chemical agent is used to disinfect the water, like chlorination.

Advantages of Rapid Sand Filtration

- It deals with raw water directly.
- It occupies less space.
- Washing of filter is easy.
- More flexibility in operation.

Chlorination of Water

Chlorination used for water purification, it kills pathogenic bacteria, it removes turbidity, color and odor.

Methods of Chlorination

Chlorine gas and chloramines are used for chlorination.

Measurements

- Orthotolidine test.
- Orthotolidine arsenite-test used.

Household Method of Water Purification

- Boiling : It kills the various microorganisms and their spores in 5 to 10 minutes.
- Chemical : By adding chlorine and other chemicals like bleaching powder, etc.
- Domestic filter : Backfield filter domestic filter used to purify the water.

PREVENTION OF AIR POLLUTION

Air pollution can cause many health disorders in human being related to respiratory system, cardiovascular system, nervous system and eye.

These problems can be prevented and controlled by taking appropriate measures for prevention and control of pollution.

Contaminated Method

This is done by various mechanical devices, e.g. in factories exhaust fans, suction apparatus and air cleaning device, etc.

Replacement Method

Replacement of coal based electricity production plants by hydroelectric power and wind powered generators are used.

Dilution Method

It can be done by extensive planting of trees and vegetation around industrial and residential area.

Disinfection of Air

This method includes mechanical ventilation which helps in reducing air bacterial density, ultraviolet irradiation for disinfecting operation theater, and infectious wards.

Legislative Method

Govt. law which has set some norms and measures to be implemented by the factories, automobiles, etc.

International Action

WHO established regional centers at various places world wide. These laboratories are set up to study the air pollution level.

Dust Control

It can be done frequently by wet dusting and wet cleaning of floors of health centers, hospitals, wards, houses, and roads, etc.

5. **Explain the following:**
   (a) Process of communication and its importance.
   (b) Methods of disinfection.
   (c) Functions of family planning clinic.

PROCESS OF COMMUNICATION AND ITS IMPORTANCE

Steps of Communication Process

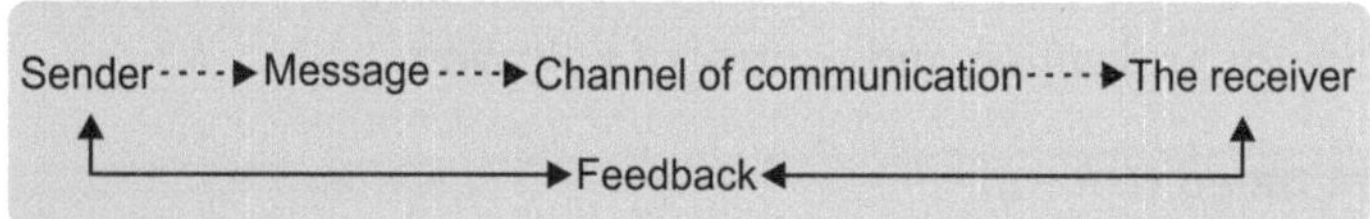

- **Sender:** Sender is the one who communicates the information.
- **Message:** The message refers to the health education information which the communicator would like to give to others.
- **Channel of communication:** It refers to the medium of giving information, e.g. radio, TV, charts.
- **Receiver:** The receivers refer to people in the community who receive the message.
- **Feedback:** It is the reaction of the community people who received the message.

Importance of Communication

- To understand and exchange ideas
- To interpret and explain to the people
- To improve interpersonal relationship
- To provide proper and prompt community services

- To change the behavior of the people
- To provide knowledge and eliminate misconcepts
- To prevent confusions or complications.

METHODS OF DISINFECTION

Definition

Killing of infectious agents outside the human body by direct exposure to chemical or physical agents.

Types of Disinfection

- **Concurrent disinfection:** The application of disinfective measures as soon as possible after the discharge of infectious material from the body of an infected person.
- **Terminal disinfection:** The application of disinfective measures after a patient died or has been removed from the hospital.
- **Prophylactic disinfection:** Boiling of water, pasteurization of milk, washing hands with soap and water are examples of prophylactic disinfection.

Various Methods of Disinfection

1.	Natural	• Sunlight • Air	
2.	Physical	• Dry heat • Moist heat • Radiation	Burning, hot dry air Boiling, steam pasteurization
3.	Chemical	• Liquids • Solids • Gases	Phenol, cresol, alcohol formation, chlorine bleaching powder, Formaldehyde, ethylene

FUNCTIONS OF FAMILY PLANNING CLINIC

The following services are available to those who visit the family planning clinics:

- MCH services (antenatal, postnatal, infant, and toddler care) through regular clinics sessions. During these sessions, education and motivation for family planning are also undertaken.
- Those who have completed their family size (2 children) are motivated to adopt for a terminal method of family planning.

- Those who visit to postpone the arrival of their next child are advised spacing methods with emphasis on oral pill or copper T-insertion.
- The IUD insertions are done daily at the clinic.
- Vasectomies are performed at the clinics attached to primary health centers and district hospital.

6. Write short notes on any (three)
   (a) Breastfeeding
   (b) Health team
   (c) Prevention of anemia
   (d) Disease cycle.

BREASTFEEDING

Breast milk is most appropriate food for a child until age of 18 to 24 months of age.

Advantages of Breastfeeding

- It is the best natural food for the baby.
- It protects the baby from infections.
- It is always clean and sterile.
- It is available 24 hours.
- It requires no preparation.
- It is free of cost.
- Available at required temperature, no need to boil.
- It creates bonding between mother and child.
- It helps parents to space their children.
- It is natural contraceptive method.
- It prevents from infectious diseases to both mother or child.

Problems in Breastfeeding

- Emotional problems, shock, worry, anxiety
- Flat nipples
- Angered breast (swollen)
- Sore or cracked nipples
- Painful tender breast
- Congenital defect
- Premature baby.

HEALTH TEAM

Definition

A health team is a group of persons who work together to promote better health in the community.

Characteristic of Health Team

- Teams have an objective.
- Health teams follow rules.
- Team members are cooperative.
- Teams organize themselves to achieve their objectives.

Health Personnel in Primary Health Center Team

- Medical officer
- Block extension educator
- Health assistant (male and female)
- Health worker (male and female)
- Health guides.

The medical officer is the leader of the health teams at the PHC level. By working alone he cannot meet the health needs of the people in the community. But by using a team of health personnel, he can provide more and better health services.

The job responsibility of other members is laid down by ministry of health and family welfare.

PREVENTION OF ANEMIA

Anemia due to Iron Deficiency

- The diet should be well-balanced and should provide adequate amounts of all dietary essentials including iron.
- In case of adults and adolescents, ferrous sulfate tablets 4 times a day.
- In case of weaned of infant 0.2 g ferrous sulfate thrice daily.

Anemia due to Folic Acid Deficiency

- Provide well-balanced diet.
- Folic acid 5 mg once daily and ferrous sulfate tablets 0.2 gm thrice daily for 10 days to adult.

Pernicious Anemia due to Vitamin B_{12} Deficiency

- Provide well-balanced diet.
- Vitamin B_{12} should be administered by injection twice a week for 2 weeks and then once a week till the anemia is cured.

After the anemia is cured, the subject should receive 1,000 micrograms of vitamin B_{12} by injection once in two months to prevent reoccurrence of the disease.

DISEASE CYCLE

The course of most communicable diseases is marked by certain stages. These are:

- **Incubation period:** This is the time interval between the entry of the disease-causing agent in the body and manifestation of clinical signs and symptoms.
- **Prodromal period:** This is a short period ranging from 1 to 4 days. Signs and symptoms not clear, clinical diagnosis is not usually possible.
- **Fastigium:** This represents the height of the disease. Sign and symptoms are clear-cut. The patient goes to bed, clinical diagnosis is possible.
- **Defervescence:** The patient begins to feel better, the body defense (Immunity) begin to respond.
- **Convalescence:** The patient's recovery is established, he is improving fast.
- **Deinfection:** The patient recovers from illness.

Community Health Nursing
December 2008

Time: 3 Hours **Maximum Marks: 75**

Note: *Attempt all the questions. All questions carry equal marks.*

1. Describe the characteristics of a healthy individual. **1×15=15**

Or

What are the uses of epidemiology?

2. Discuss in detail about waterborne diseases and their prevention. **1×15=15**

Or

Discuss in detail about airborne diseases and their prevention.

3. What are the various health education agencies in the state? **1×15=15**

Or

Discuss the role of a nurse as a health educator.

4. Describe diseases caused due to deficiency of proteins and vitamins. **1×15=15**

Or

Describe diseases caused due to deficiency of carbohydrates and minerals.

5. Write short notes on any three of the following: **3×5=15**

a. What are energy-giving foods?

b. Barriers in communications.

c. Health effects of noise.

d. Family welfare services.

e. Levels of prevention of diseases.

SOLVED QUESTION PAPER 2008

1. Describe the characteristics of a healthy individual.

Or

What are the uses of epidemiology?

CHARACTERISTICS OF A HEALTHY INDIVIDUAL

- A healthy individual is well-adjusted in every environment.
- He has a sense of personal worth and feels secure in group.
- He is able to face and solve the problem.
- He is free from conflicts and frustration.
- He feels comfortable about himself.
- He is physically healthy, has good sleeping, adequate weight, good complexion, bright eyes, sound breath, normal B and P and pulse.
- He is able to think and take action.
- He knows his own motives and desires and desires of others.
- He lives in the reality rather than fantasy.
- He has good confidence and self-esteem.
- He shows interest in job.
- He is not suffering from any mental problem.
- He has good intellectual function such as thinking, memory, perception, etc.
- His all body parts function properly.
- He has developed a philosophy of life that gives meaning and purpose to his daily activities.
- He has a variety of interests and generally lives a well-balanced life of work, rest and recreation.
- He has the ability to get enjoyment or satisfaction out of his daily routine job.
- He shows emotional maturity in his behaviors. He is able to control emotions such as fear, anger, love, jealousy and expresses them in a socially desirable manner.

Or

USES OF EPIDEMIOLOGY

Presently, the use of epidemiology is mainly confined to the following areas:

- **To study historically the rise and fall of disease in the population:** The first use of the epidemiology relates to this aspect, i.e. study of the history of disease in human population. It helps to find out the health problems and make an action plan for future.

- **Community diagnosis:** One of the uses of epidemiology is community diagnosis. It referes to the identification and quantification of health problems in the community in terms of mortality and morbidity rates and ratio. By quantification of health problem, we set down priorities in disease control and prevention.
- **Planning and evaluation:** Planning is essential in limited resources. In planning,it includes planning facilities for medical care (number of hospital beds required for patient with specific disease, health man power), planning facilities for preventive services (e.g. screening program, immunization, provision of sanitary services) and planning for research.

  Evaluation is equally important in epidemiology. It is used to find out the effectiveness of action taken.
- **Evaluation of individual's risks and chances:** One of the important tasks of epidemiology is to make a statement about the degree of risk in a population. Epidemiology is used to find out risk and causative factor of disease. The risk of bearing a mongolian child and of some hereditary disorders are classical examples of evaluating individual's risk and chances.
- **Syndrome identification:** Epidemiological investigation is used to define and refine syndrome.
- **Completing the natural history of disease:** The epidemiologist by studying disease patterns in the community in relation to agent, host and environment factors, is in a better position to fill-up the gaps in the natural history of disease than the clinician.
- **Searching for cause and risk factors:** It is used to identify the cause of disease, e.g. epidemiological study shows that rubella is the cause of congenital defects in the newborn, cigarette smoking is a cause of lung cancer; exposure of premature babies to oxygen is the cause of retrolental fibroplasias, etc.
- **Strategy formulation:** Epidemiology plays an important role in strategy formulation for disease control program and improves program efficiency and effectiveness in controlling and eradication of disease much more complex than their prevention or treatment.

2. Discuss in detail about waterborne diseases and their prevention.

Or

Discuss in detail about airborne diseases and their prevention.

WATERBORNE DISEASE AND THEIR PREVENTION

Man's health may be affected by the intake of contaminated water either directly or through food and by the use of contaminated water for personal hygiene. The water-related diseases may be classified as follows.

Biological agents	Those caused by infective agent
1. Viral	Viral hepatitis A, E, poliomyelitis, rotavirus diarrhea in infants.
2. Bacterial	Typhoid and paratyphoid fever, bacillary dysentery, *E. coli*, diarrhea, cholera.
3. Protozoal	Amoebiasis, giardiasis
4. Helminthic	Hydatid disease
5. Leptospiral	Weil's disease

Those due to the presence of an aquatic host:

Snail	Schistosomiasis
Cyclops	Guinea worm, fish tapeworm

Chemical

Chemical pollutants may affect man's health not only directly but also indirectly by accumulating in aquatic life used as human food. Other problems associated with water are:

- Dental caries due to presense of high fluoride
- Shigellosis, trachoma, conjunctivitis, ascariasis, scabies.
- Malaria, filaria these are due to accumulation of dirty water near house which gives breeding place to mosquito.

Prevention

One of the preventive measures is to purify water. Before drinking and adding in food, the water should be purified.

There are many methods which are used to purify the water and make it in drinkable form. The main and most common approaches which are used to help decontaminate the water are:

- Filtration
- Disinfection
- Boiling
- Health education

These methods are used every-where, even in houses:

Filtration

Now in market variety of filters available. It is mechanical device which makes the water pure by destroying the infective agents and other impurities from the water.

Disinfection

All water supplies are disinfected by using some chemicals like chlorine, alum, etc.

Boiling

Boiling is simple and cheapest method of water purification. It is easily used in home. Boiling for 5 to 10 minutes kills most of the microorganisms.

Health Education

Health education plays an important role in prevention of waterborne diseases.

- Provide education to people about methods of water purification and about diseases which are transmitted by contaminated water.
- Advise the people to protect the drinking water source from insects and animal contamination.
- Advise the mother about boiling of water and its use in care of infant diarrhea disease.

Or

AIR POLLUTION CAN AFFECT BY TWO WAYS

Health Aspects

The health effects of air pollution are both immediate and delayed.

Immediate Effect

On respiratory system, resulting in acute bronchitis. If air pollution is intense, it may result in immediate death by suffocation.

Delayed Effect

The delayed effects most commonly are chronic bronchitis, lung cancer, bronchial asthma, emphysema and respiratory allergies.

Social and Economic Aspects

The includes destruction of plant and animal life, corrosion of metals, damage to building, cost of cleaning, maintenance and repairs.

Some other diseases spreading by air are:
- Respiratory tract irritation
- Bronchial hyperactivity
- Impaired lungs defense
- Bronchiolitis
- Lung cancer
- Cough
- Broncho-constriction
- COPD
- Asthma
- Impaired neuropsychological development in children.

PREVENTION AND CONTROL OF AIR POLLUTION

Air pollution can cause many health disorders in human beings related to respiratory system, cardiovascular system, nervous system and eye. These problems can be prevented and controlled by taking appropriate measures for prevention and control for pollution.
- **Contaminated method:** This is done by various mechanical devices, e.g. in factories exhaust fans, suction apparatus, air cleaning device, etc. are used for a cleaning of air before discharge into the atmosphere.
- **Replacement method:** Pollution producing substances and processes are replaced with non-polluting substances and processes. Replacement of coal-based electricity production plants by hydroelectric power and wind powered generators.
- **Dilution method:** It refers to reducing pollutants in the air which can be done by extensive planting of trees and vegetation around industrial and residential area.
- **Disinfection of air:** This method includes mechanical ventilation which helps in reducing air bacterial density, ultraviolet radiation for disinfecting operation theater and infectious wards.
- **Legislative method:** Government law which can set some norms for precautionary measures to be implemented by the factories, automobiles, etc.
- **International action:** WHO established regional centers at various places world-wide. These laboratories are set up to study the air pollution level.

- **Dust control:** It can be done frequently by wet dusting and wet cleaning of floors of health centers, hospital, houses and roads, etc.

3. What are the various health education agencies in the state?

Or

Discuss the role of a nurse as a health educator.

VARIOUS HEALTH EDUCATION AGENCIES IN THE STATE

Government has a responsibility for the health education of the general public. The government of India established a central health education bureau at Delhi in 1956 to promote and coordinate health education work in the country. Many state governments in India now have other agencies. Some of them are:

- Directorate of Advertising and Visual Publicity
- Press Information Bureau
- The All India Radio (AIR)
- TV.

These are active in health education work. At the international level, there is the International Union for Health Education, with headquarters in Paris, whose main task is to promote the creation of national committees and societies for health education.

These all services are helpful in providing health education and awareness on various topics to the people, e.g.

- Nutrition
- Maternal and child health
- School nutrition program
- National control and eradication program
- Support services related to child nutrition
- Immunization
- Prevention and control of communicable diseases
- Wellness policy
- Vector control information.

Various methods are used to spread health education to the people, e.g.

- **Mass media:** TV, radio, newspapers, posters, films, cinema, flash cards, charts, black boards, seminars, role play.
- These all methods are useful for state in providing information and education to the people.
- Nowadays mass media is very effective because people come in influence of media very easily.

Aims of Health Education

- To ensure that health is valued as an asset in the community.
- To equip the people with skills, knowledge and attitudes to enable them to solve their health problems by their own actions and efforts.
- To promote the development and proper use of health services.

Principles of Health Education

- Interest
- Participation
- Comprehension
- Communication
- Motivation
- Reinforcement
- Learning by doing
- Good human relationship.

Or

ROLE OF A NURSE AS A HEALTH EDUCATOR

Health education at primary level is the responsibility of a nurse to help in bringing change in health behavior which promotes and protects health.

In Health Education, Contents Include

- Personal hygiene
- Healthy habits
- Environmental sanitation
- Nutrition
- Mother and child health
- Family welfare
- Mental health
- Health education for specific protection including immunization, protection from occupational and environmental hazards:
  - The community health nurse should communicate with the people in such a way to bring changes in health behavior and lifestyle that promote their health.
  - The community health nurse should be irrespective of her designation and place of work. It is very important for her to understand the various aspects of practice of health education and training.

- The community health nurse should include various methods for successful health education such as lecture, discussion, demonstration, case study, pamphlets, etc.
- The community health nurse has to use various health education aids/materials to make the learning more effective. Materials include auditory aids, visual aids, audiovisual aids and media.
- The community health nurse should consider following factors while she plans for health education such as the time, place and method.
- The community health nurse while planning and implementing health education may come across various constraints such as organizational support, equipment supplies, time, and place.

4. Describe diseases caused due to deficiency of proteins and vitamins.

Or

Describe diseases caused due to deficiency of carbohydrates and minerals.

EFFECTS OF PROTEIN DEFICIENCY

- Deficiency of protein in adult
- Loss of weight
- Reduced subcutaneous fat
- Anemia
- Susceptibility to infection
- Frequent loose stools
- General lethargy
- Delay in healing of wound
- Cirrhosis of liver
- Edema and ascites.

Deficiency of Protein During Pregnancy

Premature birth, stillbirth, low birth weight baby.

Deficiency of Protein during Infancy and Childhood

- Protein energy malnutrition (PEM). It is most commonly found in children between six months and three years of age, e.g. marasmus, kwashiorkor, mental retardation, stunted growth and development.
- The PEM occurs due to inadequate intake of food both in quantity and quality. Kwashiorkor is more common than marasmus in India.

Clinical Features of Kwashiorkor and Marasmus

Clinical features	Kwashiorkor	Marasmus
• Weight	Below normal, may marked by edema	Very much below normal
• Muscles	Thin (upper arm)	Very thin (upper arm)
• Edema of feet and legs	Present	Absent
• Skin	Stretched flaking skin, pale patches	Wrinkled skin
• Hair color and texture	Brighter than in others and reddish and brittle often loose	Normal color but softer than others
• Stool	Often loose	Sometimes loose, constipated
• Appetite and behavior	Poor appetite, looks miserable or irritated weak cry	Usually accepts food offered. Still but looks anxious
• Diarrhea	Often	Sometimes
• Anemia	Sometimes	Sometimes
• Vitamin deficiency	Usually found	Sometimes found

Kwashiorkor and marasmus are disease with serious consequences, because they can cause illness and death, retarded physical growth and affect mental development of the child.

Treatment

Balanced diet is treatment of protein deficiency disease. The diet usually consists of skimmed milk powder, sugar, cooked cereals and banana fat also introduced in diet. Vitamins deficiency is corrected by Vitamin supplements.

DEFICIENCY DISEASE DUE TO VITAMINS

Vitamins A

- **Night Blindness:** Inability to see in dim light.
- **Xerophthalmia:** Means dryness of the. Eye white portion of eye become dry.
- **Bitot's spots:** These are brownish, triangular, raised foamy patches seen on the white portion of the eye.
- **Keratomalacia:** The cornea (black portion) of eye becomes soft and loses its transparency.

Treatment

It is treated by well-balanced diet and supplemented with Vitamin 'A':

Vitamin D Deficiency

Rickets in young children. It is characterized by growth failure, bone deformity, muscular hypotonic, convulsion due to hypocalcemia. Milestones of development such as walking and teething are delayed.

Osteomalacia

It means softening of the bones. It mainly occurs in pregnancy and lactation. Due to deformity of the pelvis, normal delivery of baby becomes difficult.

Treatment

- Educating parents to expose their children regularly to sunlight.
- Periodic dosing of young children with Vitamin D.
- Well-balanced diet.

Vitamin E Deficiency

- Reproductive failure
- Hemolysis of red blood cells
- Muscular dystrophy.

Vitamin K Deficiency

Blood clotting time is prolonged due to prothrombin content in blood.

Vitamin C Deficiency

Scurvy

Signs and symptoms of scurvy:

- Loss of appetite
- Listlessness
- The infant cries when its legs and arms are moved
- Swelling is observed at the ends of long bones
- Hemorrhage occurs under the skin
- Gums are swollen and spongy
- Convulsion may occur
- General weakness.

Vitamin B_1 Deficiency

Beriberi, Wernick's encephalopathy. Beriberi occurring in infants is called infantile beriberi.

Signs and Symptoms

- Loss of appetite
- Tingling and numbness of the legs and hand
- Wasting of muscle and difficulty in walking.

Deficiency of riboflavin

Angular stomatitis, soreness of tongue, redness and buring sensation in the eyes, dermatitis:

- **Deficiency of niacin:** Pellagra which is characterized by soreness of the tongue, pigmented scaly skin and diarrhea.
- **Deficiency of pyridoxine:** Skin lesions, glossitis, convulsion in children.
- **Deficiency of B_{12} cyanocobalamin:** Pernicious anemia.
- **Deficiency of folic acid:** Anemia.

Deficiency of all these vitamins treated by proper intake of diet with all nutrients and treatment of underlying signs and symptoms.

Or

DISEASES CAUSED DUE TO DEFICIENCY OF CARBOHYDRATES AND MINERALS

The main sources of carbohydrates are:

- Starch
- Sugar
- Cellulose

Deficiency of carbohydrate causes constipation and it serves a fuel for the production of energy in the body but if fiber is less in diet, the body shows weakness and not able to walk in energetic manner; excess of carbohydrate also causes problem in the body, that is diabetes.

Deficiency disease caused by minerals:

Effects of Calcium Deficiency

- Decreased rate of growth
- Negative calcium balance
- Loss of calcium from bone leading to the development of osteoporosis
- Hyperplasia
- Hyper-irritability and tetany leading to death.

Effects of Phosphorus Deficiency

- Weakness in bones
- Difficulty in formation of teeth and bones
- Effect on metabolism.

Effects of Sodium Deficiency

Deficiency of sodium causes muscle cramps.

Effects of Iodine Deficiency

Deficiency of iodine leads to enlargement of the thyroid gland in the neck, a condition known as goiter. Prevention of goiter is by distribution of iodized salt throughout the country.

Effects of Fluorine Deficiency

Deficiency of fluorine causes dental caries.

Effects of Potassium Deficiency

It causes weakness and muscular paralysis.

Effects of Magnesium Deficiency

Depression, muscular weakness, vertigo, convulsions.

Effect of Iron Deficiency

It causes anemia in all age groups.

Effects of Zinc Deficiency

- Skin disorder
- Alopecia (loss of hair)
- Growth retardation
- Anemia
- Degenerative change in male and femail reproductive system.

Treatment

Treatment of these all disorders is by adequate diet with proper amount of carbohydrates and minerals. Take mineral supplementary also.

5. Write short notes on any three of the following:
   a. What are energy giving foods?
   b. Barriers in communications.
   c. Health effects of noise.
   d. Family welfare services.
   e. Levels of prevention of diseases.

ENERGY-GIVING FOODS

Food rich in carbohydrates and fats are energy-giving foods. Included in this category are eggs, cereals, roots dried fruits, sugars and fats. Cereals contain fair amount of proteins, minerals and certain Vitamins. All cereals contain starch and some incomplete protein. To achieve higher biological value of protein, the cereals must be consumed with pulses. Whole grain cereals contain thiamine and cellulose. Polished grains are of poor nutritive value than whole grains.

Other sources like oils, fats, sugar and jaggery supply calories, i.e. one gm provides nine calories and essential fatty acids. Unsaturated fatty acids are better for consumption than the saturated fatty acids and they pose minimal risk for diseases like hypertension, cardiovascular disorders and obesity, etc. Refined oils are rich in Vitamin A and D. Saturated fatty acids are good source of Vitamin A and D but should be used less. Sugar and jaggery provide enough calories, i.e. 1 gm supplies 4 calories.

BARRIERS IN COMMUNICATION

These may be:
- **Physiological:** Difficulties in hearing or expression.
- **Psychological:** Emotional disturbance, nervousness, fear, anxiety, etc.
- **Environmental:** Noise invisibility.
- **Cultural:** Customs, beliefs, religion, attitudes and level of knowledge.

HEALTH EFFECTS OF NOISE

The effects of noise exposure are of two types: Auditory and non-auditory:

Auditory

- **Auditory fatigue:** It may be associated with side effects such as whistling in the ears.
- **Deafness:** Deafness which may become permanent if the noise exposure is too high.

Non-auditory Effects

Interference with speech, inability to concentrate, loss of speech, disturbance of sleep, accidents in industries, physiological changes in the body, e.g. rise in blood pressure.

FAMILY WELFARE SERVICES

The scope of the family welfare services has become very broad. It includes the following services:
- Maternal and child health care
- Treatment of sterility
- Marriage counseling and guidance
- Premarital education
- Sex education
- Nutrition and home economics.

Because of urgent need for reduction in birth rate, emphasis is now being placed more on the MCH and family planning activities and other facets of the program are being built-up gradually.

The services provided under family planning activities are:
- Clinic services
- Domiciliary services
- **Community services:** They include family planning surveys, identification of community leaders, educational activities, motivational efforts, maintaining adequate supplies, organizing special campaigns.
- Supervisory responsibilities of the nurse.

LEVELS OF PREVENTION OF DISEASES

There are three levels of prevention:
1. Primary prevention
2. Secondary prevention
3. Tertiary prevention

Primary Prevention

Primary prevention can be defined as action taken prior to the onset of disease which removes the possibility that a disease will ever occur. The specific interventions are:
- Health promotion
- Specific protection

Health Promotion

We can prevent a number of diseases such as cholera, typhoid fever, tuberculosis and nutritional disease by promoting health of the individual and community.

Specific Protection

We prevent some specific diseases by specific measures, e.g. six killer diseases by immunization. Vitamin A deficiency by Vitamin A prophylaxis, etc.

Secondary Prevention

It may be defined as action which stops the progress of disease and prevents complication. The specific interventions are:

- Early diagnosis
- Adequate treatment

We do not have vaccines to prevent all diseases but early diagnosis and adequate treatment is only cure of that disease.

Tertiary Prevention

When the disease reaches to advance level, it is still possible to prevent. This level of prevention is called tertiary prevention.

Tertiary prevention is defined as all measures available to reduce or limit impairments and disabilities and restore the functions of individual to optimum level. The specific interventions are:

- Disability limitation
- Rehabilitation

In rehabilitation, following aspects are included:

- **Functional rehabilitation:** Restoration of functions
- **Vocational rehabilitation:** Restoration of the capacity to earn a livelihood
- **Social rehabilitation:** Restoration of family and social relationship
- **Psychological rehabilitation:** Restoration of personal dignity and confidence.

Community Health Nursing
October 2007

Time: 3 Hours ***Maximum Marks: 75***

Note: *Attempt all questions and their parts in continuity.*

1. Define the following terms: **5×1=5**

(a) Epidemiology
(b) Malnutrition
(c) Wholesome water
(d) Sewage
(e) Adulteration

2. Fill in the blanks: **5×1=5**

(a) Night blindness is caused by the deficiency of vitamin ……..
(b) …… is classified as body-building food.
(c) 1 gram of fat yields ….. calories.
(d) Deafness is caused by ….. pollution
(e) Typhoid is a ….. borne disease.

3. Write down the following: **5×3=15**

(a) Objectives of community health nursing practice
(b) High-risk families
(c) Purposes of home visiting
(d) Principles of cooking
(e) Modes of disease transmission

4. Describe as under: **5×3=15**

(a) Qualities of community health nurse
(b) Functions of under-five clinic
(c) Various types of records
(d) Small family norms
(e) Characteristics of healthy individual.

5. (a) Write down the immunization schedule for 0.5 years age group children. **5×3=15**

(b) Explain the barriers of communication.

(c) Role of nurse in the primary health care.

6. **Write short notes on any four:** **5×4=20**
   (a) Community health nursing process
   (b) Household methods of preserving and storing food
   (c) Immunity
   (d) Water pollution
   (e) Light diets.

SOLVED QUESTION PAPER 2007

1. **Define the following terms:**
   (a) Epidemiology
   (b) Malnutrition
   (c) Wholesome water
   (d) Sewage
   (e) Adulteration

EPIDEMIOLOGY

Epidemiology is concerned with the pattern of disease occurrence in human population and of the factors that influence these patterns.

MALNUTRITION

It is a condition, which occurs when the body does not get the proper kind of food in the amounts needed for maintaining health.

WHOLESOME WATER

The water which is free from harmful pathogenic organisms, chemical substance, pleasant to taste, fit for domestic use.

SEWAGE

Sewage may by defined as water from a community containing solid and liquid excreta derived from houses, street-washings, factories and industries.

ADULTERATION

It is malpractice to substandardized the food stuff by mixing, concealing the quality, misbranding, giving false labels and addition of toxicants.

2. **Fill in the blanks:**
   (a) Night blindness is caused by the deficiency of vitamin ....
   (b) ...... is classified as body building food.
   (c) 1 gram of fat yields ..... calories.

(d) Deafness is caused by ….. pollution
(e) Typhoid is a ….. borne disease.

FILL IN THE BLANKS

(a) Night blindness is caused by the deficiency of **Vitamin A**.
(b) **Protein** is classified as body building food.
(c) 1 gram of fat yields **9 calories**.
(d) Deafness is caused **by noise** pollution.
(e) Typhoid is a water-borne disease.

3. **Write down the following:**
   (a) Objectives of community health nursing practice
   (b) High-risk families
   (c) Purposes of home visiting
   (d) Principles of cooking
   (e) Modes of disease transmission.

OBJECTIVES OF COMMUNITY HEALTH NURSING PRACTICE

The main objectives of community health nursing practice include the following:

- Health promotion
- Health maintenance
- Prevention of illness
- Restoration of health.

Health Promotion

Health promotion is to increase the level of understanding and the expectations of families, groups and communities to cope with health and illness problems. In this way, include modifying (change) the health practices of people, increase knowledge and developing understanding of normal growth and development.

Health Maintenance

It involves continuous assessment of both individual and community to ensure that they continue to function at the same level.

Prevention of Illness

Prevents the community from illness, e.g. it is to maintain and increase level of immunization in the family to prevent occurrence or reoccurrence of the disease.

Restoration of Health

It is to help the patient or community person in returning to an optimum state of health and well-being.

HIGH-RISK FAMILIES

These days WHO developed and promoted new approach to identify high-risk families in the population by some defined criteria. Criteria for the high-risk families are:

Biological Situation

- Age groups, e.g. infants, elderly, etc.
- Sex, e.g. female in reproductive age group.
- Physiological problem during pregnancy, e.g. cholesterol level, high blood pressure in family, obesity, etc.
- Other health conditions.

Physical Situation

Physical situation such as rural, urban area, living conditions, overcrowding environment problem, e.g. water pollution, unhygienic conditions, overpopulation, over-pollution, etc.

Socioeconomic and Cultural Situation

Families include which have poor socioeconomic conditions such as:

- Social group.
- Family distruption, education, housing
- Customs, habits, behavior
- Lifestyle and living standard of family.

In order to reduce high-risk families, primary prevention plays an important role. In this health education plays important role. Early detection and treatment of disease and immunization.

All these steps taken by the government are beneficial to the community persons and may reduce the number of high-risk families.

PURPOSES OF HOME VISITING

- It is a routine part of a planned visiting program by a community health personnel.
- It helps to investigate the source of infections disease.

- To do follow-up on some problem identified in the health center, school, industry or hospital.
- To assess the nutritional and immunizational status and environmental hazards.
- To give health education to the individual, family, and community.
- To supervise and guide other health workers.
- To carry out simple nursing care and procedure in the home situation.
- To carryout procedure for prevention of diseases and promotion of health of the members of the family.

PRINCIPLES OF COOKING

Cooking is an art which changes the flavor, texture, appearance and taste of food and makes it in easily digestible form.

The basic principles are:

- Food must not be overcooked or undercooked to prevent the loss of essential nutrients.
- It sterilizes the food by killing microorganism, ova and eggs.
- It gives veriety to the food; same patterns of cooking may lead to selection of some nutritious foods.
- Excessive use of condiments like salt and red pepper may lead to common problem like hypertension, piles, etc.
- Good cooking increases the acceptability of food.
- It must be done in hygienic place. Handling and stocking of food must also be done in some hygienic place.
- Cooking area must have a sufficient distance from sanitary place.

MODES OF DISEASE TRANSMISSION

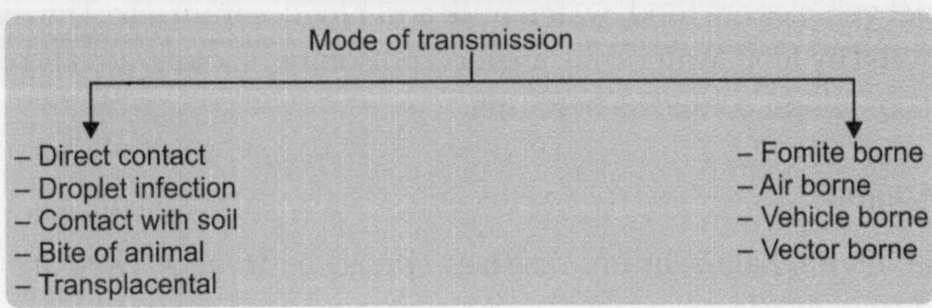

Direct Transmission

Direct Contact

Some diseases transmitted directly from person to person by direct contact such as touching, kissing, etc. Diseases spread by direct contract are AIDS, rabies, etc.

Droplet Infection

Fine drops of secretion from infected person spread disease, e.g. by sneezing, coughing, spitting, singing and talking, etc. and diseases spreads through droplet transmission are common cold, diphtheria, tuberculosis, etc.

Inoculated Directly in Skin or Mucosa

When the infectious agent inoculated directly into skin, e.g. dog bite. Rabies is caused by bite of rabid animal.

Transplacental Transmission

Some diseases spread by placenta from mother to fetus, e.g. AIDS, It is also called vertical transmission of disease.

Indirect Transmission

Fomites borne

Fomites are articles other than food and drinking. The articles which are infected by patient and used by healthy person, cause disease. Articles, e.g. pencil, books, clothes, etc.

Airborne

The infectious agent which comes out from infected person by different ways, if inhaled by healthy person, it causes infection.

Vehicle Borne

The chief vehicles are food, water, milk and blood, serum, etc. The diseases transmitted by food, water, milk are food poisoning, cholera, etc. and disease spreads by blood contact is hepatitis.

Vector borne

Malaria, fileria, kala-azar are diseases spread by insects. They are called vector borne diseases.

4. Describe as under:

(a) Qualities of community health nurse
(b) Functions of under-five clinic
(c) Various types of records
(d) Small family norms
(e) Characteristics of healthy individual.

QUALITIES OF COMMUNITY HEALTH NURSE

- She has coordination with the fellow men.
- She should be honest and loyal.
- She should be disciplined and obedient.
- She should be alert and intelligent in observation.
- She should be technical minded.
- She should be adjustable everywhere with every situation.
- She should be confident.
- She should have resourcefulness.
- She should be able to save time, material and energy.
- She should be sympathtic and empathic.
- She should have courtesy and dignity.
- Intelligence and common sense.
- She should have patience and sense of humor.
- She should have generosity.
- She should have good physical and mental health.
- She should have gentleness and quietness.

FUNCTIONS OF UNDER-FIVE CLINIC

Care in Illness

In this health care and treatment to sick children should be provided, 10 to 90%, care in illness can be provided by nurse. So they need to be given proper training and delegation of responsibility.

Preventive Care

- **Immunization:** Immunization is the birth right of every child. The goal of this is to immunize all children against major infectious diseases.
- **Nutritional surveillance:** The food supplements are often an intergral part of child health care. It includes mid-day meal program and vitamins for prophylaxis.
- **Health check-up:** This is undertaken every 3 to 6 months. The child health care provides a checklist for these examinations.
- **Oral rehydration therapy:** The mothers are taught oral rehydration therapy in case the child has diarrhea.
- **Family planning:** Family planning is an important component of child welfare.
- **Health teaching:** Health education is necessary for each part of services and it binds them altogether.

Growth Monitoring

One of the basic activities of the under-five clinic is growth monitoring, i.e. to weigh the child periodically at monthly intervals during the first year; every 2 months during the second year and every 3 months thereafter upto the age of 5–6 years.

VARIOUS TYPES OF RECORDS

Types of Records

- **Cumulative or continuing records:** Cumulative records containing information which is collected in a period of time of each patient in different situations. When completed cumulative records: include whole history of patient, e.g. immunization history, school health records also included.
- **Family records:** All the records which relate to members of one family should be placed in single family folder. It is useful for health worker to know the health status of full family in one time.
- **Clinical records:** It is used in the hospital investigation, special treatment and procedures are written and signed in these records.
- **Doctor order sheet:** It includes doctor order about medication, investigation, procedures, etc.
- **Nurses sheet:** The nurse records the treatment and procedure carried out by the nurses, and observation made on the patient.

Other Records

TPR chart, lab report sheet, diet sheet, intake output chart, anesthesia chart, special treatment chart.

Some other types of records which are maintained in community settings:

- Family and village record
- Eligible couple and child register
- Sterilization
- MCH care register
- Child care register
- Birth and death register
- Subcenters/PHC/Clinical register
- Subcenters/PHC/Clinical register
- Reports of blood stain of malaria and filaria
- Monthly reports
- Daily diary, etc.

SMALL FAMILY NORMS

All efforts are made by mass communication so that all people adopt and accept the 'Concept of small family norms'.

Family size plays an important role in health of individual, community and families and whole nation.

Effects of Family Size

- **Basic human needs:** Food, clothing, shelter, education are basic need of human, if family size is big, they are not satisfied.
- **Economical needs:** Income, saving and resources may not be sufficient to meet if the family size is large.
- **Food and nutrition:** The larger family size will not be able to meet the nutritive requirements of the members of the family.
- **Socioeconomic:** Large family size results in poor socioeconomic condition of population.
- **High morbidity and mortality rate:** Large family results in high morbidity and mortality rate among mothers and children.
- **Education:** It is hard for the large family to give proper education to their children.

Advantages of Small Family Norms

- **The mother:** The mother gets more time to participate in other activities such as education, vocational training and community projects also.
- **The child:** The child will get good atmosphere for his proper physical and psychological growth and development. The child gets proper nutrition, education, parental love and care.
- **The father:** The father can provide children with better education, comfort, food, clothing recreation, etc.
- **The community:** Small size of population helps the community to provide enough facilities to the people such as water supply, schools, health care services, etc.

CHARACTERISTICS OF HEALTHY INDIVIDUAL

- A healthy individual has same insight and understanding of his motives, desires, his weaknesses and strong points.
- A healthy individual feels comfortable about himself.
- He has a sense of personal worth and feels important.
- A healthy individual is able to meet the demands of life.

- He has a sense of personal security.
- He has faith in his ability to succeed, he believes that he will do reasonably well whatever he undertakes.
- Mentally healthy person lives in a world of reality rather than fantasy.
- He has developed a capacity to tolerate frustration.
- He shows emotional maturity in his behavior.
- He is able to think for himself and can make his own decision.
- He has a variety of interests.
- He does not suffer from disorder of mental functions such as thinking, emotion, memory, etc.
- A healthy individual has capacity for hard-work.
- He is well adjusted with self and with the environment.
- He has self-control.
- He feels right towards others.
- He experiences a sense of happiness.
- He is able to solve the problems of others.

5. (a) Write down the immunization schedule for 0.5 years age group children.

(b) Explain the barrier of communication.

(c) Role of a nurse in the primary health care.

IMMUNIZATION SCHEDULE

Refer Important Theory, Q. No. 12.

BARRIERS OF COMMUNICATION

- **Psychological:** When the persons emotionally disturbed and not able to concentrate and not perceive the stimuli, not able to exchange his own ideas.
- **Physiological:** When the person has any physical problem like difficulty in hearing.
- **Environment:** Environment like noise in the area where any person talks to another, e.g. school building near the main road and near railway line disturbs concentration of speaker and listener. Other environmental causes are invisibility due to dim light or glare.
- **Cultural:** Cultural factors such as illiteracy, customs, beliefs, language, social class also become barriers in communication.

ROLE OF A NURSE IN THE PRIMARY HEALTH CARE

- Community health nurses works with population, community, family on individual basis.

- Assessing the health status of individuals and communities.
- Mobilizing community involvement.
- Providing integrated health care including the treatment of emergencies and making referrals.
- Maintaining epidemiological surveillance.
- Training and supervizing health workers.
- Collaborating with other development sectors.
- Monitoring progress in primary health care.
- She focuses on assessment of the impact of the socioeconomical and cultural factors affecting health.
- She works in school where primary goal is health education and disease prevention.

6. Write short notes on any four:

(a) Community health nursing process
(b) Household methods of preserving and storing food
(c) Immunity
(d) Water pollution
(e) Light diet.

COMMUNITY HEALTH NURSING PROCESS

Introduction

It is systematic method for assessing health status, diagnosis of health needs, formulating a care plan, implementation and evolution of plan.

Purpose

- To assess the health needs of people
- To maintain patient's optimal well-being

Steps

The nursing process consists of the five phases:

- **Assessment:** This phase assesses the health needs of people and collects information by using various methods such as questioning, interview or nursing history.
- **Diagnosis:** It is a clinical judgment about individual, family or community problems. During this phase, analysis and interpretation of data which is collected during assessment phase take place.

- **Planning:** In this phase the intervention or nursing care planned to minimize or correct and prevent the problems which are identified in the nursing diagnosis.
- **Implementation:** It refers to carry out action, which is planned to solve the problems. It includes procedures, tasks, practices which are actually implemented by nurse.
- **Evaluation:** It is ongoing process which determines the extent (degree) to which goals of health care are achieved or which to be modified.

Advantages of Nursing Process

- It helps to identify the health problems.
- It helps in communicating nursing therapies and other related actions.
- Helps to define specific nursing responsibility.

HOUSEHOLD METHODS OF PRESERVING AND STORING FOOD

Preservation

It is a technique in which variety of foods are stored for a long period *Refer Paper 2009, Q. No. 4(a).*

IMMUNITY

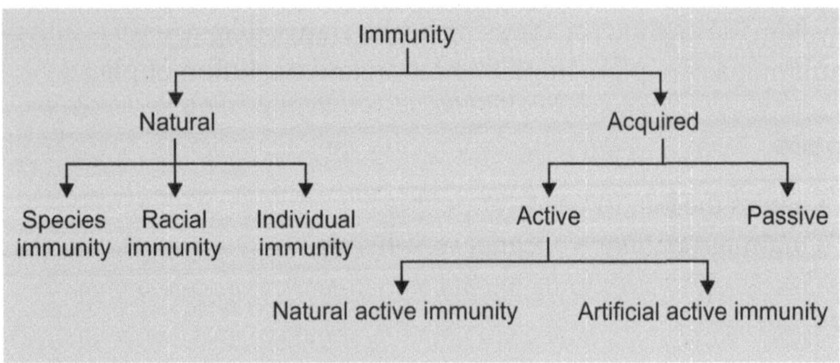

- It is power of body to fight against infection.
- **Natural immunity:** Natural immunity or inherited immunity is that immunity which the individual inherits or possesses by his genetic make-up.

It is also divided into 3 types:

1. **Species immunity:** It is total resistance shown by all members of particular species. It is due to physical and biochemical differences, e.g.

Human beings are resistant to plant pathogens and many animal pathogens.

2. **Racial immunity:** Within a species, there may be marked social difference in resistance to infection.
3. **Individual immunity:** Every individual has own different immunities to fight against infection.

Acquired Immunity

This may be two types active and passive immunity:

- **Active immunity:** It is the immunity which a person develops as a result of infection by pathogenic organisms or their toxic products. It also has two types:
  1. Natural active immunity
  2. Artificial active immunity
- **Passive immunity:** When the antibodies produced in one person are transferred to another to give protection against a disease, it is called passive immunity.

WATER POLLUTION

One of the problems of the modern day is pollution of water supplid by man himself.

Sources of Water Pollution

- **Agriculture sources:** The use of chemicals and pesticides of all kinds in agricultural field creates the problem of ground water and surface water pollution.
- **Sewage:** This is a serious source of water pollution, which contains decomposable organic matter and pathogenic agents.
- **Industrial source:** Wastes from industries and factories, which contain toxic agents cause water pollution. It does not kill only fish, but also harms human beings.
- **Physical sources:** Heat and radioactive substances also create water pollution.

Water-related Diseases

Human being's health may be affected by the ingestion of contaminated water. The term water-related disease includes the classical waterborne diseases.

Biological (Waterborne diseases)

Viral	:	Viral hepatitis A, E, Poliomyelitis, rotavirus, diarrhea in infants
Bacterial	:	Typhoid, paratyphoid, dysentery, diarrhea, cholera
Protozoal	:	Amebiasis
Helminthic	:	Roundworm, threadworm, hydatid disease
Leptospiral	:	Weil's disease

Those due to the presence of an aquatic host:

Snail	:	Schistosomiasis
Cyclops	:	Guinea worm, fish, tapeworm

Chemical

It includes:
- Dental caries
- Cyanosis in infant
- Cardiovascular
- Trachoma
- Conjunctivitis
- Scabies.

LIGHT DIET

This diet contains all the required nutrients, especially proteins and carbohydrates. It is modified diet for therapeutic use to meet the nutritive requirements of sick individual.

Purpose

- To maintain good nutritional status.
- To correct the deficiencies which have occurred.
- To provide rest to body metabolism.

The hospital diet plays a very important role in the life of the patient. The diets which are suitable for feeding in hospital are:
- Clear fluid diets
- Full fluid diets
- Soft diet
- Light diet.

Characteristics of Light Diet

- It should be of low residue.
- It should be bland with no spices and condiments.

- Plenty of fluids to be included to maintain electrolyte balance.
- Light diet is prepared for persons suffering from fever, very ill patients who cannot chew or swallow solid food. To avoid difficulty in swallowing, fibrous food and irritating spices are not included in this diet.
- The protein content increased by adding skimmed milk powder in the soups and beverages.
- The energy content of the diet can be increased by adding cream to milk, butter/oil to cereal, dal, soups, milk, etc.
- Light diets are offered to chronic patient, pre-operatively, postoperatively, because in chronic disease, there is increase in the nutritional requirement.

Community Health Nursing
October 2006

Time: 3 Hours | **Maximum Marks: 75**

Note: *Attempt all questions and their parts in continuity.*

1. Define the following terms. **1×10=10**

(a) Disease
(b) Disinfection
(c) IMR
(d) Immunity
(e) Incubation period
(f) Motivation
(g) Cold chain
(h) Epidemic
(i) Rehabilitation
(j) Health

2. Enlist the following: **5×3=15**

(a) Basic needs of family.
(b) Household methods of water purification
(c) Water-soluble and fat soluble vitamins
(d) Uses of vital statistics
(e) Principles of primary health care.

3. Writer down the following: **5×3=15**

(a) Sources of vitamin A
(b) Water-borne diseases
(c) Characteristics of mentally healthy person
(d) Vector borne disease (Mosquitoes)
(e) Protein-energy malnutrition

4. Write down briefly. **5×4=20**

(a) Methods of family planning
(b) Balanced diet
(c) Principles of home visit
(d) Objectives of school health
(e) Immunization

5. (a) Mention the functions of food **5×3=15**

(b) Principles of recording and reporting
(c) Prevention of AIDS in community
(d) Functions of community health nurse
(e) Sources of noise

SOLVED QUESTION PAPER 2006

1. Define the following terms.

(a) Disease
(b) Disinfection
(c) IMR
(d) Immunity
(e) Incubation period
(f) Motivation
(g) Cold chain
(h) Epidemic
(i) Rehabilitation
(j) Health

DISEASE

Any deviation from normal function or complete physical or mental well-being is called disease.

DISINFECTION

Killing of infectious agents outside the human body by direct exposure to chemical or physical agents.

IMR

Infant mortality rate is defined as the number of infant deaths per 1,000 live births in one year.

IMMUNITY

It is the ability or power of body to fight against infection.

INCUBATION PERIOD

This is the time interval between the entry of the disease agents into the body and the appearance of the first sign or symptom of the disease.

MOTIVATION

It is an inner force which drives individual to a certain action. It also determines human behavior.

COLD CHAIN

It is a system of transporting and storing vaccines at the recommended temperatures.

EPIDEMIC

Epidemic means an outbreak of disease in a community in excess of 'normal expectation' derived from common source.

REHABILITATION

The process of restoring a person's ability to live and work as normally as possible after illness or injuries.

HEALTH

It is a state of complete physical, mental and social well-being and not merely an absence of disease.

2. Enlist the following:

(a) Basic needs of family
(b) Household methods of water purification
(c) Water-soluble and fat-soluble vitamins
(d) Uses of vital statistics
(e) Principles of primary health care

BASIC NEEDS OF FAMILY

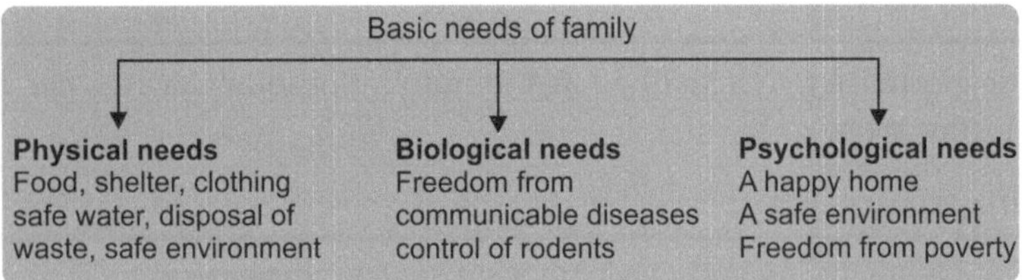

HOUSEHOLD METHODS OF WATER PURIFICATION

- **Boiling:** Boiling for 5 to 10 minutes kills full bacteria, spores, virmes and removes temporary hardness of the water.
- **Chemicals:** Commonly chemicals which are used for purification of water are bleaching powder, alum, potassium permanganate and chlorine tablets.
- **Domestic filters:** Water-purified by domestic filters such as Berkefeld filter.

WATER-SOLUBLE AND FAT-SOLUBLE VITAMINS

Fat-soluble

- Vitamin A
- Vitamin D
- Vitamin E
- Vitamin K.

Water-Soluble Vitamins

- Vitamin B complex
- Vitamin C
- Riboflavin
- Nicotinic acid
- Pyridoxine
- Pantothenic acid
- Folic acid
- Vitamin B_2
- Ascorbic acid
- Thiamine.

USES OF VITAL STATISTICS

- To measure the state of health of a community and to identify its health problems and health needs.
- For comparing the health status of one country with that of another.
- For comparing the present status with that of the past.
- For planning and health administration.
- For evaluation the progress, success or failure of health programs and services in operation.
- For research into community health problems.

PRINCIPLES OF PRIMARY HEALTH CARE

Refer Paper November 2010, Q. No. 5(a).

3. Write down the following:

(a) Sources of vitamin A.
(b) Waterborne disease.
(c) Characteristics of mentally healthy persons.
(d) Vector borne diseases (Mosquitoes).
(e) Protein energy malnutrition.

SOURCES OF VITAMIN A

- Animal sources – Butter, ghee, egg, milk
- Vegetable sources – Spinach, coriander, carrots
- Fish liver oil
- Synthetic Supplements

WATERBORNE DISEASES

Refer Paper October 2007, Q. No. 6(d) (Water-related diseases).

CHARACTERISTICS OF MENTALLY HEALTHY PERSON

Refer Paper October 2007, Q. No. 4(e)

VECTOR BORNE DISEASES

- Anopheles — Malaria
- Culex — Filaria, encephalitis
- Aedes — Yellow fever, Dengue fever, Hemorrhagic fever
- Mansonoides — Filaria

PROTEIN ENERGY MALNUTRITION

It is severe protein deficiency disease.

Signs and Symptoms

- Weakness in general health
- Swelling of body tissues due to accumulation of fluid in the tissue space
- Poor resistance

Protein starvation can result from lack of protein in diet in persons due to lack of available supplies of protein foods or through ignorance. Satisfy their hunger needs with large amount of CHO.

4. Write down briefly.

(a) Methods of family planning
(b) Balanced diet
(c) Principles of home visit
(d) Objectives of school health
(e) Immunization

METHODS OF FAMILY PLANNING

Temporary Methods

For Men

- Condom
- Withdrawal

For women

- Intrauterine devices
  - Copper T
  - Lippes loop
  - Diaphragm.

Hormonal Contraception

- **Oral pills:** Mala - D, Mala -N
- **Injectables:** DMPA, NET–EN
- Subdermal Implants (Norplant)
- Foam tablets, jelly and cream
  - Rhythm method (safe period)
  - Coitus interruptus.

Natural Method

Breastfeeding

Permanent Method

- Male sterilization, e.g. Vasectomy
- Female sterilization, e.g. Tubectomy.

BALANCED DIET

Definition

- Balanced diet is the one which consists of all the required nutrients in correct or adequate amount for proper maintenance and regulation of body functions.
- Every age group requires different level of calories, e.g.

Infant below 6 months needs 120 kcal/kg body weight.

- Infant age 6 to 12 months : 800 calories, 13 gram protein
- Preschool children : After one year of age, adding 100 kcals for every year
- During pregnancy : + 300 calories, 15 gm protein
- During lactation : + 550 calories, 25 gm protein

PRINCIPLES OF HOME VISIT

- **Need based:** Home visiting should be planned and conducted according to the needs of the people.
- **Priority based:** The home visit should be given priority according to the existing problems in the family. It may be maternal and child health services or antenatal check-up.

- **Regularity:** Home visiting should be planned at regular intervals to fulfill the identified needs.
- **Flexibility:** The community health nurse should adopt a flexible approach according to circumstances at home.
- **Scientific based:** Use scientific skill including handwashing, an inspection, etc.
- **Analysis based:** Collect background information about the home, the patient and the environment and make an objective analysis of the facts as an initial step in visiting the home.
- **Developing relationship:** Home visiting helps to establish good working relationship in the family.
- **Senstivity:** The community health nurse should be sensitive to the person feeling at the time of the visit. Listen to the family and understand the other person's point of view.
- **Evaluative:** Evaluate your own work, remember the quality of care is more important than the number of home visits. It is essential to evaluate home visits from time to time.

OBJECTIVES OF SCHOOL HEALTH

- To increase health awareness in children about health.
- To educate and guide the school children to adopt healthy habits and healthy lifestyle.
- To facilitate early diagnosis and treatment of school children in school.
- To promote interest of students in individual and community health activities.
- To work towards a total personality development of school children in all dimensions—physical, mental, social, emotional and moral.
- Growth and development.
- Controlled population.
- Group living.

IMMUNIZATION

Refer Important Theory, Q. No. 12.

5. (a) Mention the functions of food.
(b) Principles of recording and reporting.
(c) Prevention of AIDS in community.
(d) Function of community health nurse.
(e) Sources of noise.

MENTION THE FUNCTIONS OF FOOD

- Provision of energy
- Body building and repair
- Maintenance and regulation of tissue functions.

PRINCIPLES OF RECORDING AND REPORTING

- Records are written documents. It is essential that it should be written clearly, accurately, appropriately and legibly.
- All entries should be signed by the individual who writes them.
- Care should be taken not to make any error on the record.
- Records should be written in chronological order with date and time.
- Use only standard abbreviations.
- Records not given to any strange person.
- It is not sent outside without authority.
- It is written in language which is understandable by every health worker.

PREVENTION OF AIDS IN COMMUNITY

Education

Until a vaccine or cure of AIDS is found, the only present treatment is education. Education to people to make life-saving choices, e.g. avoiding indiscriminate sex, using condoms.

- One should also avoid the use of shared razors and toothbrushes.
- Education to the drug users, they should not share needle and syringes.
- Education to the women who are HIV positive, they should not conceive pregnancy because the infection transmition is from mother to fetus. For this purpose, use various educational material, and mass communication, etc.

Prevention of Blood-borne HIV Transmission

People in high-risk groups should be discouraged for donation of blood. All blood should be screened for HIV-1 and HIV-2 before transfusion. Strict sterilization practices should be used in hospitals and clinics if possible avoid use of disposal syringes and avoid injection unless they are absolutely necessary.

Specific Prophylaxis

At present there are no vaccines or cure for treatment of HIV infection/ AIDS. AZT (Zidovudine) antiviral chemotherapy is useful to rescue the immune system.

Primary Health Care

Because of its wide ranging health implications, AIDS touches all aspects of primary health care, including mother and child health, family planning and education.

FUNCTIONS OF COMMUNITY HEALTH NURSE

Administration

The nurse is responsible for the day-to-day assignment of the nursing staff and supervising the health personnel.

Communication

She develops good working relationship with members of the health team, related agencies and the community for effectiveness of health services.

Nursing

She provides comprehensive nursing care to individual and families. This includes care of mother and child, antenatal, intranatal, postnatal, child care, immunization, nutrition and family planning.

Teaching

She uses knowledge, skill and simple teaching aids for training of the health workers and she participates in student training programs.

Research

She participates in all research activities related to community improvement.

SOURCES OF NOISE

There are many sources of noise:

- Domestic sources-transistors, radio and TV.
- Automobiles and railways.
- Factories and industries.
- Aircraft, etc.

Community Health Nursing
September 2005

Time: 3 Hours **Maximum Marks: 75**

Note: *Attempt all questions.*

1. Define the following: **10×1 = 10**

(a) Family (b) Perception
(c) Emotion (d) Health
(e) Intelligence (f) Mental health
(g) Food additives (h) Nutrition
(i) Vital statistics (j) Sewage

2. (a) Write down the classification of food. **5+5=10**
(b) What are the functions of proteins?

3. (a) What are the principles of primary health care? **5+5+5=15**
(b) Write the methods of refuse disposal.
(c) Explain the methods of group teaching.

4. (a) Define health education. **1+5+4=10**
(b) Write down the principles of health education.
(c) Discuss the role of community health nurse in family welfare services.

5. (a) What are the principles of home visiting? **5+5+5=15**
(b) Explain the procedure of bag technique.
(c) What are the preventive and control measures of malaria?

6. Write short notes on any three of the following: **5×3=15**

(a) Under-five clinics
(b) Protein calorie malnutrition (PCM)
(c) Referral system
(d) Prostitution
(e) Prevention of AIDS.

SOLVED QUESTION PAPER 2005

1. Define the following:

(a) Family
(b) Perception
(c) Emotion
(d) Health
(e) Intelligence
(f) Mental health
(g) Food additives
(h) Nutrition
(i) Vital statistics
(j) Sewage

FAMILY

It is defined as 'a group of individuals that have blood relation, living together and eating from a common kitchen, living under one room'.

PERCEPTION

Perception is the interpretation of sensory stimuli which reach the sense organs and brain, interpretation gives meaning to sensation and we become aware of the objects.

EMOTION

Gates defined emotions as the episodes in which the individual is moved or excited.

HEALTH

According to WHO 'Health' is a state of complete physical, mental and social well-being and not merely an absence of disease or infirmity.

INTELLIGENCE

According to Thorndike

Intelligence is the ability to give responses that are true.

MENTAL HEALTH

Mental health is described as a healthy mind. But it cannot be described without physical, social, spiritual health. Mental health is a part of general health. It requires balance between the body, mind, spirit and the environment in which a person lives.

FOOD ADDITIVES

A substance added to food to improve its appearance and increase its nutritional value. When substandardized food quality by malpractice, it is called food adulteration.

NUTRITION

Nutrition is the intake of food, considered in relation to the body's dietary needs.

VITAL STATISTICS

It is the numerical description of birth, death, abortion, marriage, divorce, adoption, etc.

SEWAGE

It is defined as the water from a community, houses, street, washing, factories and industries which contains solid and liquid excreta.

2. (a) Write down the classification of food.
(b) What are the functions of proteins?

CLASSIFICATION OF FOOD

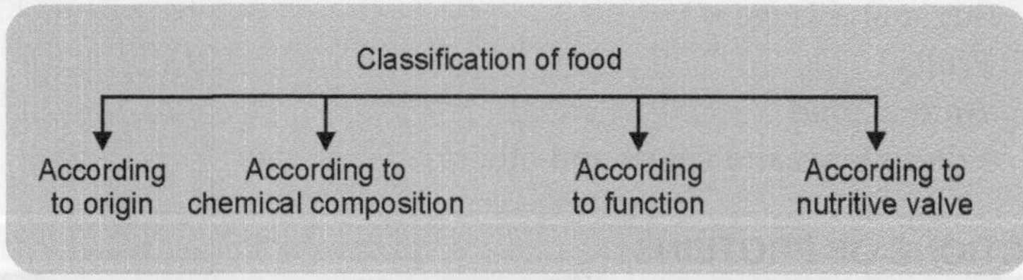

1.

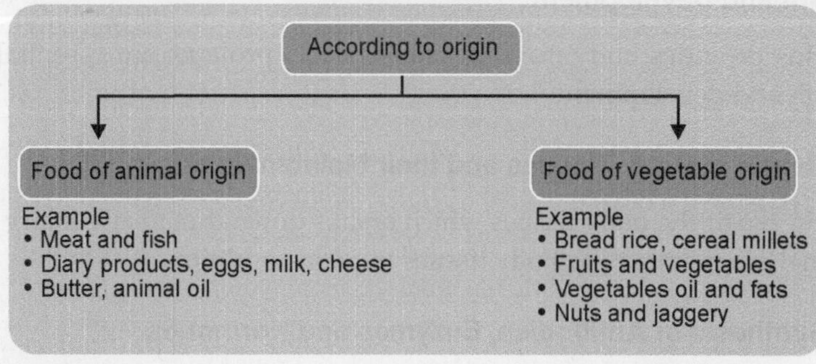

2.

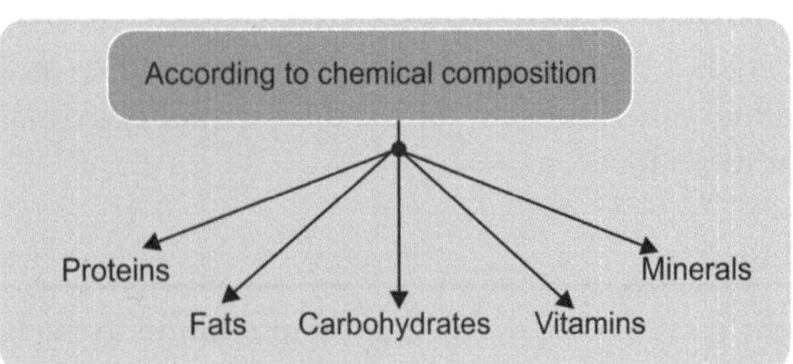

3.

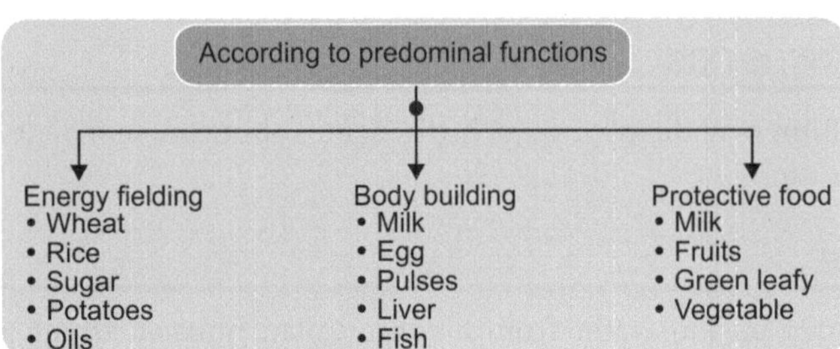

4. **According to Nutritive Value**
    - Cereals
    - Pulses
    - Vegetables
    - Nuts
    - Sugar and jaggery
    - Fruits
    - Animal food
    - Condiments and spices and others.

FUNCTIONS OF PROTEINS

Growth and Development

Proteins provides body building material. So proteins are essential for growth and development.

For Repair of Body Tissues and their Maintenance

Protein repair the body tissues which breaks down due to any injury and they help in maintaining body tissues in good condition.

For Synthesis of Antibodies, Enzymes and Hormones

Antibodies, enzymes and hormones contain protein and these all are essential for body to protect from infection.

3. (a) What are the principles of primary health care?
(b) Write the methods of refuse disposal.
(c) Explain the methods of group teaching.

PRINCIPLES OF PHC

Refer Paper November 2010, Q. No. 5(a).

METHODS OF REFUSE DISPOSAL

- **Burning:** The best method for refuse disposal is burning or incineration. Hospital refuse is best disposed by burning but before burning remove glasses and tin material.
- **Dumping:** It is a simple method of refuse disposal by dumping in low lying area where after some time it changes in manure and it is very useful for vegetation.
- **Controlled tipping:** In this made 3 feet deep pit and refuse dispose in this pit. After 3 to 6 months it changes in manure by bacterial action at the end of 6 months it is opened and removed mannure for agriculture use.
- **Composting:** When refuse and human excreta is placed with refuse in 3 feet deep pits, It is called composting. Spread of alternative layers of excreta and refuse.

METHODS OF GROUP TEACHING

- **Lectures:** It is most popular method of group teaching. In this communication mostly one-way—the people are only passive listeners. A lecture does provide basic information on the subject but it may fail to change the health behavior of the people.
- **Group discussion:** It is a two-way teaching method people learn by exchanging views and experiences for group discussion required not less than 6 people and there should be a group leader who lead the people, and sum-up the discussion in the end.
- **Films and charts:** These are mass media of communication. They can be of value in educating small group.
- **Demostration:** It is an important technique of health education. We show people how a particular thing is done by using a tooth brush, bathing a child, feeding an infant, etc.
- **Seminars and conferences:** In this method a large group takes part. Each one presents his point of view on a given subject.

- **Symposium:** It is series of speeches on a selected subject. Each person presents about the subject briefly.
- **Workshop:** The workshop consists of a series of meeting and divided into small groups. Hearing takes place in a friendly, happy, democratic atmosphere under expert supervision.

4. (a) Define health education.
(b) Write down the principles of health education.
(c) Discuss the role of community health nurse in family welfare services.

HEALTH EDUCATION

Health education has been defined as a process which effects changes in the health practice of people and in the knowledge and attitude related to such changes.

PRINCIPLES OF THE HEALTH EDUCATION

- **Interest:** The health education should be related to interest and needs of the people. Because without interest people will not learn.
- **Participation:** It is better than passive learning personal involvement help in good learning. In this, both group and educator participate.
- **Comprehension:** The teaching should be within the mental capacity of the people. We must know the level of understanding, education and literacy level of people.
- **Communication:** In health education, we should never use words which are strange and new to the people. Use simple words which are familiar to people.
- **Motivation:** Stimulation or awakening the desire is called motivation. In health education, we try to motivate individuals and groups to accept new ideas.
- **Reinforcement:** Few people do not learn the new in a single period, repetition at intervals is necessary.
- **Learning by doing:**
  Learning is an active process:
  - If I hear I forget
  - If I see I remember
  - If I do, I know
- **Good human relation:** The health educator must be kind and sympathetic people must accept him as their real friend.

ROLE OF A NURSE IN FAMILY WELFARE SERVICES

Administrative Role

The community health nurse's has to participate and organize family welfare programs at a national, regional and community level as an administrator.

Functional Role

The community health nurse functions include assisting doctor in prenatal, postnatal, and biological tests.

Supervisory Role

As a supervisor, community health nurses should encourage their staff to participate actively in family welfare program. She organizes work for other health workers, professionals and auxilliary nursing personnel.

Educational Role

By using her knowledge and skill, she educates the community and patient about family life, family planning, methods of regulating fertility, etc.

Role in Research

She participates in research activities for improvement in family welfare services.

Evaluation Role

Evaluation is an important part of planning and nursing services in relation to use of family welfare services.

5. (a) What are the principles of home visiting?
(b) Explain the procedure of bag technique.
(c) What are the preventive and control measures of malaria?

PRINCIPLES OF HOME VISITING

Refer Paper October 2006, Q. No. 4(c).

PROCEDURE OF BAG TECHNIQUE

Refer Paper 2013, Q. No. 5(b).

PREVENTIVE AND CONTROL MEASURES OF MALARIA

Preventive Measures

- Avoid collection of water near the house places and other parts of the city or village.
- Sanitary improvement, such as filling all the pits, ponds, pools, etc. to eliminate the breeding places of mosquito and larvae.
- If insecticides are not available, then use oil for spraying in living and sleeping quarters.
- Use synthetic insecticides, e.g. DDT, BHC, etc.

Anti-larval Measures

- **DDT:** It is effectively used in little amount, e.g. 5 to 10 precent oily solution used for spraying.
- **Paris green:** It is mixed with 100 parts of slaked lime, fine road dust, saw dust, sea stone, etc. and is sprayed.
- **Anti-adult measures:** In this method mosquitoes mainly in the houses, building, etc. are sprayed.
- **Protect against bite of mosquitoes** by applying repellents. Cover the body with clothes, using mosquito nets and screening houses.

Measures for Personal Protection

- The use of topical ointment (odomos)
- Use of mosquito nets
- Use of mesh doors and windows.

Control Measures

- Isolate patient in screened room or use mosquito net to prevent spread of this disease.
- Investigate source of infection, contacts and find out history of previous attack of malaria from the person.
- Report about the case to the health authority immediately.
- Infected places should be disinfected by spraying effective insecticide.
- Survey should be done to find out case in endemic area.

6. Write short notes on any three of the following:

(a) Under-five clinics

(b) Protein calorie malnutrition (PCM)

(c) Referral system

(d) Prostitution
(e) Prevention of AIDS

UNDER-FIVE CLINICS

Refer Paper October 2007, Q. No. 4(b).

PROTEIN CALORIE MALNUTRITION (PCM)

It is the common nutritional problem in the preschoolers. It affects on growth and development of a child. Poor resistance and swelling of body tissues due to accumulation of fluid in the tissue space. There is one main disease under this category as explained below.

Kwashiorkor

This disease is caused by deficiency of calories:

- Here child looks thin, skiny due to severe muscle wasting
- Weight loss is more
- The child's mental status is intact
- Appetite is good with no skin, hepatic and hair change.

This illness develops soon after weaning when the child no longer receives protein supply from his mother's milk.

REFERRAL SYSTEM

Referral system means transfer of the patient from one health institution to another for better health care services. A good referral system is an essential

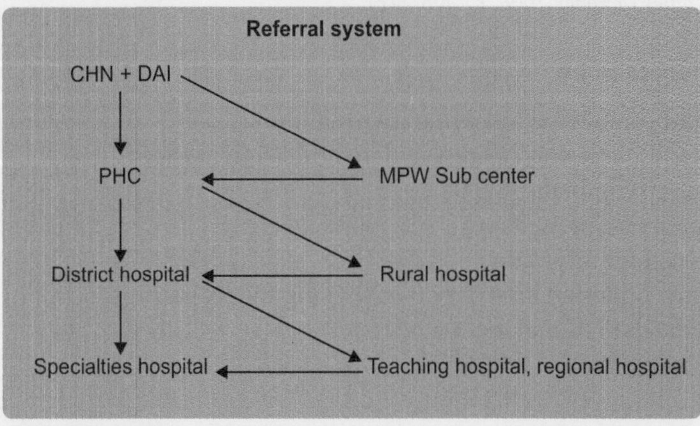

component of health care system. As more and more paramedical workers are employed in the health industry, it becomes necessary to establish a sound referral system.

PROSTITUTION

Prostitution is a social evil. It is a social problem in most urban areas.

Causes

- Changes in environment
- Breakdown of family relations
- Parental quarrels
- Want of affection
- Poverty
- Low IQ
- Low moral standards
- Ill-treatment by parents, husband or relatives
- Death of parents or husband.

Prevention

- Education plays an important role to control some of these problems by disease education to the parents about care of own children.
- Education to the parents about the basic needs of the children according to growth and development.
- The government of India Act in 1956 known as 'The suppression of Immoral Traffic Act in Women and Girls' bans prostitution.

PREVENTION OF AIDS

Refer Paper October 2006, Q. No. 5(c).

References Slips

It should contain the following information:

- Patient name and address and identification number
- Present complaints
- Treatment given, if any
- Reason for referral
- Name of designation of person making the referral
- Name of PHC making the reference
- Date and time of reference.

Community Health Nursing
September 2004

Time: 3 Hours | ***Maximum Marks: 75***

Note: *Attempt all the questions and their parts in continuity.*

1. Define the following: **2×5=10**
- (a) Vegetarian
- (b) Habits
- (c) Calorie
- (d) Defence mechanisms
- (e) Society

2. (a) What do you understand by food preservation and food storage? **10+10=20**
(b) List down various methods of cooking.

3. (a) Write in detail the functions of primary health center. **10+10=20**
(b) Discuss the qualities of community health nurse.

4. (a) List family planning methods. **5+10=15**
(b) Discuss in detail national family planning program.

5. Write any two of the following: **5+5=10**
- (a) Well-baby clinic
- (b) Immunization schedule
- (c) Methods of cooking.

SOLVED QUESTION PAPER 2004

1. Define the following:

(a) Vegetarian
(b) Habits
(c) Calorie
(d) Defence mechanisms
(e) Society

VEGETARIAN

The person who only eats vegetable food is called vegetarian.

HABITS

Habits is an accustomed way of doing things.

CALORIE

It is defined as the amount of heat required to raise the temperature of 1 kg of water by 1 degree celsius at a specific pressure.

DEFENCE MECHANISMS

Defence mechanisms are the techniques or mechanisms used by an individual to handle tension to reduce anxiety or resolve conflicts.

SOCIETY

A society may be defined as a group of people who have lived together long enough to become organized and are considered as a unit more or less distinct from human units.

2. (a) What do you understand by food preservation and food storage?
(b) List down various methods of cooking.

PRESERVATION

A technique in which variety of foods are stored for a long period is known as preservation.
Refer Paper 2009, Q. No. 4(a).

VARIOUS METHODS OF COOKING

Refer Important Theory, Q. No. 3, Related to Nutrition.

3. (a) Write in detail the functions of primary health center.
(b) Discuss the qualities of community health nurse.

FUNCTIONS OF PRIMARY HEALTH CENTER

Definition

Primary health center provides essential health care made universally accessible to individuals and families in the community by means acceptable to them, through their full participation and at a cost that the community and country can afford.

Functions

- **Heath education:** Health education is an integral part of all health services and all health personnel responsible for educating people about improving their own health, immunization and prevention or control from communicable diseases.
- **Promotion of food supply and proper nutrition:** The responsibility of PHC is to provide essential health services. These include proper supply of food and nutrition to overcome nutritional deficiency disease among children and mothers.
- **Maternal and child health care, including family planning:** In PHC, community health nurse is assigned to carry out maternal and child health services. In this include care of mother during antenatal, intranatal and postnatal care, care of children and distribution of family planning methods.
- **Immunization:** Immunisation facilities provided by PHC against six killer diseases for children and tetanus. For pregnant, women immunisation is done by health worker of PHC.
- **Adequate safe water supply and basic sanitation:** In PHC, the sanitary inspectors and health workers are responsible for sanitation. They guide the people about sanitary latrine, sewage disposal and chlorination of water.
- **Prevention and control of local endemic diseases:** In India, government has launched various program for control and eradication of these endemic diseases. These programs are implemented by PHC for the health of people.
- **Appropriate treatment of common diseases and injuries:** Primary health center provides treatment against common diseases and injuries which are not serious and make referral of serious injuries.

- **Provision of essential drugs:** Some drugs for minor problems are available in PHC.

QUALITIES OF COMMUNITY HEALTH NURSE

- She coordination with the fellow workers.
- She should be honest and loyal.
- She should be disciplined and obedient.
- She should be alert and intelligent in observation.
- She should be technical minded.
- She should be adjustable everywhere with every situation.
- She should be confident.
- She should be resourcefulness.
- She should save time, material and energy.
- She should be sympathetic and empathetic.
- She should have courtesy and dignity.
- She should have intelligence and common sense.
- She should have patience and sense of humor.
- Generosity.
- Good physical and mental health.
- Gentleness and quietness.

4. (a) List family planning methods.
(b) Discuss in detail national family planning program.

LIST OF FAMILY PLANNING METHODS

Refer Paper October 2006, Q. No. 4(a).

NATIONAL FAMILY PLANNING PROGRAM

- In 1953, family planning program was launched by union ministry of health and family welfare.
- During the first and second Five-year Plans program focus way given on four components education, services, training, research.
- During the third Five-year Plan the program was recognized, after the publication of the 1961 census result, which showed higher growth rate than expected.
- In 1966, a full fledged department of family welfare was set-up.
- During fourth Five-year Plan, top priority was given to the program.
- In the fifth Five-year Plan the approach was to integrate family welfare services with those of mother and child health services.

- In 1983, the national health policy was approved by Parliament.
- In 1985–86, universal immunization started.
- Various other programs implemented during seventh Five-year of Plan.
- In 1992, during eighth Five-year Plan program integrated child survival and safe motherhood program.
- During the ninth Five-year Plan, the RCH program integrated all the related program of the eighth plan.
- The overall objective of this program is to stabilize the population with the requirement of national development.

5. Write any two of following:

(a) Well-baby clinic

(b) Immunization schedule

(c) Methods of cooking.

WELL-BABY CLINIC (UNDER-FIVE CLINIC)

In this clinic offers the best combination of curative, preventive and promotive care services.

Aims and Objectives of Well-Baby Clinic

Refer Paper 2007, Q. No. 4(b).

IMMUNIZATION SCHEDULE

Refer Important Theory, Q. No. 12.

METHODS OF COOKING

- **Boiling:** Cooking in water at 100°C is called boiling.
- **Simmering:** Cooking below the boiling point is about 84°C is called simmering.
- **Steaming:** This is cooking by the heat of direct steam, e.g. pressure cooker.
- **Frying:** This is of 2 types IM shallow frying is suitable for cooking food like eggs, dosa; deep frying is suitable for making puri, pakora, etc.
- **Roasting:** Food is smeared with a little fat and exposed directly to heat or flame.
- **Baking:** Baking is cooking food by dry heat. It is done in a hot air oven.
- **Broiling or grilling:** It is cooking by direct dry heat, it can be done either in a grill or heavy pan or direct on flame.

Effects of Cooking on Food

Carbohydrates	Gelatinization will occur
Protein	Coagulates at 60°C, boiling hardens albumin and globulin
Fats	Melts during cooking
Vitamins	Some loss during cooking
Minerals	These are not affected by cooking
Fruits	Cooking destroys most of Vitamin B
Egg	Albumin coagulates at 65°C
Green leafy vegetables	Thiamine and Vitamin C are partially destroyed by cooking.